# Praise for
## *The Mindfulness for Warriors Handbook*

"This is a book that will save lives. *Mindfulness for Warriors* is a work of major importance that offers practical approaches to self-care and serenity for our first responders. Our military veterans, firefighters, police, dispatchers, paramedics, doctors, and nurses are at the front lines of our society and a vital part of every community. Kim Colegrove's marvelous book is an essential read for these brave people."

**—Louise Harmon, author of *Happiness from A to Z***

"Kim Colegrove has one audacious goal—to save the first responders who put their own lives on the line for others every day. Through candid memoir, insightful interviews, and informed advice, *Mindfulness for Warriors* offers practical tools for first responders and the people who love them. Colegrove artfully blends her account of the heart-wrenching loss of her husband with her wisdom from decades of meditation practice and her hope to find a solution to the trauma dynamic that rips first responders from the world. Colegrove's firsthand experience watching lives change for the better authorizes her to make this bold claim: mindfulness can save lives. She's seen it and tells us how it's done. Hers is a message you won't want to miss."

**—Nita Sweeney, meditation teacher, writing coach, and award-winning author of *Depression Hates a Moving Target***

"*Mindfulness for Warriors* is an outstanding book I will be giving to a lot of people. My father was a Marine who came back from war and became a fireman. I loved how brave Dad was, but I also sensed, behind his tough exterior, he was hiding a lot of pain. He was a stoic who forged on doing his very important work but at a high personal cost. He and so many like him serve our communities and deal with extreme stress on a daily basis, often without any way to process the pain and PTSD they are suffering. Kim Colegrove's book is an invaluable tool to help the helpers. Her mindfulness practices and meditation techniques offer much respite, relief, and calm to anyone who picks up this book."

**—Becca Anderson, author of *Prayers for Hard Times* and *Real Life Mindfulness***

"Kim Colegrove survived unspeakable grief, and, rather than becoming bitter and broken herself, she honed a fierce and relentless compassion that seeks well-being for those who protect and serve. This book, and the PauseFirst Project, offer accessible tools for everyday use. In its pages, you will find solid strategies and proven practices for coping with stress and trauma in work and in life. *Mindfulness for Warriors* is a must-read for veterans, first responders, and all who walk the way of the warrior."

**—Rev. Roxanne Pendleton, MDiv, CYT 200, advisor, Trauma Informed Care, and author of *Laughing Again: A Survivor's Guide to Healing Depression***

"While many of us might not consider ourselves warriors. In truth, we are. Especially if, as the author writes, 'your life or work involves helping, saving, and rescuing others....' From time to time, we become rescuers for our kids, partners, friends, family, or co-workers. This groundbreaking book, therefore, is a must-read since it touches all of us. It not only documents the lives of others who needed help, but it also provides very grounding solutions for dealing with and overcoming life's challenges."

**—Allen Klein, author of *Embracing Life After Loss***

"The pain of trauma that first responders suffer from is finally being recognized, and *Mindfulness for Warriors* shows the path to healing. Kim Colegrove shares her heart-wrenching story of the loss of her husband to suicide, why it happened, and effective keys to recovery through mindfulness meditation. *Mindfulness for Warriors* is a welcome guide not only for first-responders and their loved ones, but anyone who suffers from trauma."

**—Rev. Connie L. Habash, LMFT, author of *Awakening from Anxiety: A Spiritual Guide to Living a More Calm, Confident, and Courageous Life***

# THE
# MINDFULNESS
## FOR
# WARRIORS
## HANDBOOK

# THE
# MINDFULNESS
## FOR
# WARRIORS
## HANDBOOK

### Stress Reduction, Trauma Recovery,
### and Resilience Building
### for First Responders

## KIM COLEGROVE

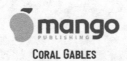

**mango**
PUBLISHING

CORAL GABLES

Published by Mango Publishing Group, a division of Mango Media Inc.

Cover, Layout & Design: Megan Werner

For permission requests, please contact the publisher at:
Mango Publishing Group
2850 S Douglas Road, 2nd Floor
Coral Gables, FL 33134 USA
info@mango.bz

For special orders, quantity sales, course adoptions and corporate sales, please email the publisher at sales@mango.bz. For trade and wholesale sales, please contact Ingram Publisher Services at customer.service@ingramcontent.com or +1.800.509.4887.

The Mindfulness for Warriors Handbook: Stress Reduction, Trauma Recovery, and Resilience Building for First Responders

Library of Congress Cataloging-in-Publication number: has been requested
ISBN: (pb) 978-1-68481-439-8 (e) 978-1-68481-440-4
BISAC category code HEA055000, HEALTH & FITNESS / Mental Health

Printed in the United States of America

This book is dedicated to
David M. Colegrove

# CONTENTS

## Part 1
## THE WARRIOR

## Part 2
## THE WEIGHT

**Part 3**
# THE WISDOM

# Publisher's Note

# LET'S HELP THOSE WHO DO MUCH FOR US

My dad, Walter, was a Marine who enlisted right before his eighteenth birthday. Growing up on a farm in Kentucky didn't prepare him for what he saw on the battlefields of World War II. He went to war as a boy and came back a man, albeit one with a lot of shock and pain because of what he saw and experienced in Japan. This was, of course, before the concept of Post-Traumatic Stress even existed. PTSD was recognized by advocates, physicians, military veterans, and activists after lengthy activism on behalf of Vietnam veterans, many of whom came home from war in deep distress. Physical wounds are very grave, and layering on psychological wounds makes a return to regular life nearly impossible. One of my uncles, a naval officer, used to say, "You can leave the war, but the war might not leave you." Veterans are the first responders of our nation; they defend our country and rush into battle to defend all of us.

Other first responders also rush in wherever help is needed and go where others fear to tread. Firefighters, police officers, EMTs, emergency room staff, and many more folks deal with high stress situations where others' lives depend on them. Those who retired from these roles don't magically release their trauma when they leave the job. In fact, it is often compounded, because they no longer have their friends and coworkers to talk and let off steam with.

No one knows this more than author Kim Colegrove. Her beloved husband, Dave, was a law enforcement officer who retired after dedicating decades to his career. He retired and, after three months to the shock of his family and friends, took his own life. He quit the job, but the job didn't quit him. All that stress and pain, built up over years, had no outlet. He made a choice, one we never want a loved one to make.

This book is intended to help the helpers.

This book is intended to provide outlets.

This book provides tools to deal with and heal the trauma.

Kim Colegrove also made a choice. Though devastated with a crushing grief, she dedicated the rest of her life to helping other first responders. Kim and her trainers offer techniques to first responders to regain their mental health, find their center, and return to living life fully. She founded Pause First Academy, where she and former first responders share and teach these brave people how to regain their resiliency. She also wrote a book, *Mindfulness for Warriors*. When the proposal first came in, I immediately thought of my dad and how he suffered in silence, like so many of these stoics do. By the time I reached the second page of the proposal, I knew I wanted to publish what I saw as a very important book. I remember telling my fellow Mangos that this would be a book that will save lives. And it has.

I could not be more proud of this expanded edition of Kim's book, which includes a moving story of one of those lives. We have also included a resource section for warriors, filled with more help for those who save our lives on a daily basis, just by doing their jobs.

If you know a veteran or a retiree or have a loved one serving our country who can use some stress relief, gift them this book. I have gifted copies to my local police, firehouse, and also a dispatcher who would start tearing up when she talked about some of the calls she gets. Dispatchers are first responders too.

I want to take the opportunity to thank Kim for her courage in turning her pain into action. You inspire me, Kim. Brava!

We would love to hear from you too, and I invite you to contact me directly at my email below. I hope this book helps you, and I wish you all the best and a life filled with awesomeness.

Be well,
**Brenda Knight**
Publisher, Mango Publishing Group
Brenda@MangoPublishingGroup.com

# Preface

In December of 2022, I attended my publishing company's annual holiday get-together online. This is an opportunity for fellow authors, my editor/publisher Brenda Knight, and others from Mango Publishing to come together, share, and celebrate.

Our facilitator, Sherry Richert Belul, author of *Say It Now* and host of Mango's weekly Heart Wisdom author panels, kicked off the festivities by asking everyone to tell a positive story about their book, their year, or whatever they felt like sharing with the group. I decided to talk about something I had experienced just a few days earlier during an in-person training.

On the Saturday before this holiday celebration, three fellow Pause First Academy instructors and I presented a full day of training for first responder retirees and those who anticipate retiring in five or so years. The workshop, *Navigating Retirement: Creating a Path to Purpose, Fulfillment, and Wellbeing,* is intended to help people plan for and process the mental and emotional aspects of retirement.

Each attendee received a copy of the original version of this book, *Mindfulness for Warriors: Empowering First Responders to Reduce Stress and Build Resilience.* On breaks, a few people asked me to sign their copy or approached me to chat or ask questions. During one break, a man approached me with the book in his hand, and I assumed he wanted a signature. I was not prepared for what he had to say.

He told me he appreciated receiving a copy of the book and shared that he had already read the book. "Your book saved my life," he said.

I was caught off guard, and I wasn't sure how to respond. Tears filled his eyes as he continued, "I had a suicide plan, and I was ready to execute that plan. And then your book came onto my path, and I changed my mind."

An intense feeling filled my body, like a little shockwave or an adrenaline surge. I was flooded with emotions. However, this wasn't the first time I'd heard the words, *Your book saved my life*.

I can't describe the depth of humility and gratitude that fills me when I hear these words. It feels like I'm being given an important gift, along with a card that says, "With this gift comes great responsibility."

I take my work seriously, because I have come to know how many people across first responder professions are suffering due to the weight of the work. And I know all too well from my own experience how bad things can get when people refuse to, or aren't afforded the opportunity to, deal with the crushing pressure of that weight.

The sharing of my workshop story sparked a new level of interest within my publishing company. In the early months of the following year, they gave me the green light on a second book and decided to retitle, enhance, and rerelease *Mindfulness for Warriors* under a new program called *Books that Save Lives*.

I felt some hesitation around this idea in the beginning. My initial concern was that people would buy the book, realize they'd already read it, and feel duped. My publisher addressed my concerns and assured me we would take precautions to avoid that issue by making it abundantly clear that the new book was a reprint of *Mindfulness for Warriors*, with some additional information and a new resource directory.

The more I thought about it, the more it made sense to retitle and rerelease the book. For one thing, this would be an opportunity to use a new subtitle to describe more directly what the book offers: stress reduction, trauma recovery, and resilience building. And I liked the idea of freshening up the cover art to help the book appeal to a wider audience.

In the final section of the book, I define and describe meditation and mindfulness and offer simple ways to experiment with these evidence-based practices. But that's just one segment. The first two thirds of the book offer my personal story of loss, and the narrative of nine veterans and first responders who share their stories. The storytelling combined with an examination of trauma, mental health, and suicide are the headliners. I, and the people I interviewed, share our experiences and suggest resources, ideas, tools, and skills to help guide and support others through their journey of stress reduction, trauma recovery, resilience building, and healing.

Ultimately, I'm glad we made the updates, and I'm thrilled with the final product. So, without further ado, I present to you, *The Mindfulness for Warriors Handbook*. And I'd like to introduce you to Keith, the man who told me my book saved his life, which inspired this redesign, and paved the way for a second book.

Up until a couple of months before this rerelease was set to happen, I wasn't sure who the man was that approached me at that retirement training. I was so taken aback by his comment that I felt a little *Twilight Zone*-ish in the moment, but, after a bit of detective work, I was pretty sure his name was Keith.

One week after the in-person training, I and the rest of the training team held an optional follow-up meeting via Zoom so we could check in with attendees, find out how they were doing, and answer questions about what they had learned. Keith attended that meeting, but he didn't turn on his camera, so I couldn't confirm it was him. I was super curious, but I decided to let it go. Until it was time to write this preface.

I had Keith's email address because, also during that Zoom training, we did a prize drawing, and he won. I requested that the winner send me an email with their mailing address so I could send them the prize. (As I look back, it feels like the whole thing was kind of fated.)

I really wanted to speak to the guy from the training before writing the preface for this rerelease of my book, so I took a chance and emailed Keith and here is what I said:

> Hi Keith. I'm not sure if I have the right person or not. Did you talk to me during the workshop in Branson and share that you had already read my book? I feel terrible that I'm not sure if this was you or not, but the person who spoke with me told me my book saved his life. I was taken aback and a little shocked in that moment, and later I wished I had made a mental note of the person's name tag.
>
> If this was you, and you might be willing to speak with me, I would be most grateful. If this was you, and you prefer not to speak with me, I understand, and I'll let it go.

He quickly wrote back, confirmed that it was him, and said he would be happy to help in any way, especially if it might help other people. The rest, as they say, is history.

And now, I'd like you to meet Keith.

# • KEITH •

**Law Enforcement**

31.5 Years

Patrol Officer

Rapid Response Unit

Tactical Team/SWAT

Detective: Sex Crimes, Child Abuse, Homicide

Cold Case Sex Crimes

Property Crimes

Fire Investigation

Keith and I met for this interview via Zoom, and we spoke for around two hours. Our conversation was deep, real, and raw. He was open and honest and allowed himself to be vulnerable. I was moved to tears and goose bumps during portions of our chat. I asked him the same five questions I had asked the other warriors in my first book:

1. What is your professional background?

2. Can you share a little about some of the difficult experiences you've endured?

3. Was there a turning point?

4. Which tools have you found most useful on your journey?

5. What needs to change in these cultures to support well-being?

Here's what I learned about Keith and his over-thirty-year career as a first responder.

First of all, he was a single dad. He raised his only daughter by himself while also dealing with the intense demands of a law enforcement career. During his darkest times, his relationship with his daughter suffered, and the two were estranged for a period of time.

## Difficult Experiences

Keith ticked off a list of the usual difficult experiences most police officers endure, then moved pretty quickly to an event that occurred very early on and sort of hung over the rest of his career.

While Keith was in the police academy, he was involved in a shooting during a ride along with a veteran officer. They attempted to stop a suspicious vehicle, which led to a car chase. As they pursued the car, the driver in the passenger seat began shooting at the police car through the back window.

At some point, the car stopped. The shooter jumped out of the car and ran. The duty officer engaged in a foot chase, leaving Keith behind with the other occupant of the car. Keith remembers the shooter pointing his gun directly at him and firing, but the gun didn't discharge. Keith was shocked that he wasn't hit during all of the shooting.

He was in full academy uniform and was wearing body armor, but because he was a recruit, he wasn't allowed to carry a gun. He wasn't sure what to do without a firearm to protect himself, so he got in position behind the door of the police car, acting as if he was holding a gun. He ordered the guy to the ground, then approached him and held him down, waiting for backup, which thankfully arrived.

While he was alone with the passenger, he heard more shots fired. He later learned that the suspect had been shot by the other officer but didn't die.

As the police officers secured the scene, Keith was placed in a police car alone, for what felt like a very long time. After that, he was taken to headquarters where he was interviewed by detectives. He remembers feeling scared and confused, like maybe he was in trouble or might be facing dismissal. He wasn't released to go home until late into the night, and he had to report to the academy early the next morning.

The next day at the academy, the recruits were going through scenarios—role-playing to test decision-making and response to situations they might encounter on the job.

Afterwards, Keith was jotting down notes, completing an after-action report, and one of the academy trainers noticed his hands were shaking. The trainer asked him if he was shaken up by role-playing and Keith said no, he wasn't sure why his hands were shaking. He told the instructor that he had been in a shooting the night before while on a ride along, and he hadn't had much sleep. (Flash forward to the present, Keith now realizes he was experiencing physical symptoms caused by the traumatic experiences of the night before.)

Keith's shaking hands and mention of the shooting led to an immediate academy investigation. The next thing he knew he was in a room by himself where he had been asked to write a detailed report recounting his experience the night before. Once again, he felt worried that he was in some kind of trouble or that he might lose his job.

Ultimately, he did not get in trouble, nor was he dismissed. But that experience, and the surrounding emotion, fear, worry, and trauma, stuck with him throughout his career. He didn't dwell on these things, but he realizes now, they were always there.

Keith witnessed two other shootings early in his career, another officer-involved and one accidental shooting that occurred during a training exercise.

## Turning Point

Keith's turning point came late in his career, when he was working as a fire investigator. He started to notice he was losing the ability to emotionally disengage from cases. He felt the hard outer shell that had allowed him to conduct the investigations dispassionately was no longer there to protect him from the emotions of the work.

His point of no return was initiated by a particularly difficult fire investigation involving twin babies that died in a home fire. Keith determined that one baby had died of smoke inhalation, and the other had burned to death, and this realization hit him hard. He became extremely emotional over this case, and it haunted him like nothing before.

Keith says that's when he started to experience symptoms of severe trauma, although he didn't know much about trauma at the time. For whatever reason, that case opened a Pandora's Box of feelings, memories, and images. Things from the past started coming up. He experienced terrible nightmares, many sleepless nights, and would sometimes go three or four days at a time without any sleep.

The Mindfulness for Warriors Handbook

He began drinking heavily and drinking himself to sleep every night. He remembers episodes of uncontrollable crying while in his police car. He was losing his tolerance of citizens, and his behavior, actions, and drinking started to push his now-adult daughter away, which led to an estrangement.

It was during this time that Keith decided he didn't want to live anymore, so he set about getting his affairs in order to ensure that everything he owned would go to his daughter.

During the course of planning his suicide, Keith heard about an organization called The Battle Within, a five-day retreat in nature for first responders and veterans struggling with anxiety, depression, Post-Traumatic Stress, or a diagnosis of PTSD. He applied for the program, and the prospect of possibly getting help gave him a small glimmer of hope. He temporarily put his suicide plan on hold. He thought, *I'll try this and if it helps, maybe I won't kill myself.*

But this happened in the height of COVID, and he wasn't able to get the days off work to attend the program. However, one of the members of The Battle Within staff sent him a copy of my book, *Mindfulness for Warriors.*

Keith started reading the book immediately and says he remembers crying because he no longer felt alone. The book helped him realize that others have felt the way he had been feeling. He connected strongly with the first responders and veterans and their stories.

As a result of reading the book, Keith says, he quit drinking alcohol, started experimenting with mindfulness, and put his suicide plans on hold.

Next, his daughter started to come back around, which solidified his decision not to kill himself. He also decided to get professional help.

At first, Keith tried to hide the fact that he was in therapy from his employer. But when his therapist recommended that he seek more targeted and in-depth help from a local in-patient program for veterans and first responders with PTSD, he knew he would have to make his employer aware. He did so and then immersed himself into the program, and completed the out-patient follow-up as well.

Keith says he felt supported by his employer when he was honest about his situation and attended the program. But he also felt somewhat isolated.

He is now retired. He admits to feeling sad when he left the job. But looking back, he knows it was the right thing to do. He says retirement saved his life, and he knows it will also extend his life.

Keith has strong advice for anyone in a similar position who will listen:

> Don't wait. I waited too long, and it almost cost me my life. If you don't want your employer to know, then go get help on your own. But don't wait and let this ruin your life, because it will.

For those of you who are wondering if Keith and his daughter reconciled, they did. He's been honest with her about his struggles and his path to healing, which has helped them work on rebuilding and redefining their relationship.

## Tools Keith Has Found Most Useful

- Mindfulness
- Counseling
- EMDR Therapy[1]
- Writing and journaling

## What Needs to Change

Keith was quick to answer, "Let the stigma go." While he admits to sometimes still feeling a little embarrassed, he remembers that, prior to seeking help, he felt that asking for help was a sign of weakness, a signal he couldn't handle the job, and that he'd be viewed as a loser if he sought help.

Now, he realizes that is all part of the stigma that prevents first responders from seeking life-saving assistance with their job-related trauma.

As part of his "don't wait" message, Keith goes on to say, "First responders must be encouraged to address trauma at the time they experience it. Trying to ignore the symptoms or hold in the emotions will not work. The memories, images and feelings *will* resurface. So, people have to deal with them and process them when they happen."

"Think of it this way," he continues, "you're not going to keep running on a sprained ankle, you're going to get it looked at. You should deal with mental and emotional wounds in the same way."

Keith remains focused on healing and still attends counseling sessions. He practices mindfulness and uses writing and journaling to help him process the difficult things. He hasn't figured out what's

---

1   As a side note, Keith points out that it's crucial to find a therapist who specializes in first responder trauma and PTSD, both for counseling and EMDR Therapy.

next for him in life, so for now, he does a lot of volunteer work and continues to work on himself.

I am beyond grateful to Keith, the nine first responders and veterans who contributed to this book, and the others I am speaking with now who will be featured in my upcoming second book.

I know this will be difficult for some of you to read. It deals with heavy and sometimes emotionally triggering topics, but the information and stories provided here are important. Gone are the days of turning a blind eye to the pain and suffering of our first responders. Culture change is on the horizon, and it will usher in a whole new generation of healthy, balanced warriors, protectors, guardians, and healers!

# Foreword

This is an outstanding book I will be giving to a lot of people. My father was a Marine who came back from war and became a fireman. He saw hand-to-hand combat and was wounded by a sword on the Japanese island of Iwo Jima in World War II. Dad not only survived, he brought home the sword that nearly killed him; it was displayed proudly beside an American flag in our living room. My dad was a badass. So are first responders.

I loved how brave Dad was, but I also sensed, beneath his tough exterior, he was hiding a lot of pain. He was a stoic who forged on without complaint, doing his very important work but at a high personal cost. So many more like him serve our communities and deal with extreme stress on a daily basis, often without any relief or any way to process the pain and PTSD they are suffering. Post-traumatic stress disorder is a serious syndrome and can't be ignored. Tamping down those feelings for too long can lead to major consequences, as Kim Colegrove discovered with her husband's tragic suicide. Our first responders—police, military, firefighters, paramedics, hospital workers, dispatchers, and many more do so much to help others; more often than not, they don't get around to helping themselves. In this book, Colegrove provides marvelous tools offering renewal for these courageous people who do so much for the rest of us.

Kim Colegrove's book is an invaluable tool to help the helpers. Her mindfulness practices and meditation techniques offer much respite, relief, and calm to anyone who picks up this book.

—**Becca Anderson**, author of *Prayers for Hard Times* and *Real Life Mindfulness*

# Introduction

"To know even one life has breathed easier because you have lived. This is to have succeeded."

**—Ralph Waldo Emerson**

Here's how this whole thing started.

Me: I want to teach cops how to meditate.

Pretty much everyone else on the planet: You will never get cops to meditate.

Me: Hold my beer.

The catalyst to this work was my husband's death by suicide in 2014. I never intended to become an advocate for culture evolution in law enforcement and other first-responder professions, but here I am.

Meditation and mindfulness are personal practices that empower an individual to become familiar with and regulate the self. They are evidence-based, meaning there's research to support my mission. When you learn these skills and practice them regularly, you can use them to settle and neutralize your system—mentally, physically, and emotionally.

*Nobody* needs this information more than emergency responders—police, firefighters, EMTs, paramedics, other EMS roles, dispatchers, corrections officers, active military and veterans—and I'm also going to include social workers and other mental health professionals, clergy, ER professionals, and others in the mix. Although these would not technically fall under the heading of "first responder," their experiences of stress, trauma, and secondary trauma mirror those of first responders.

The technical definition of a first responder is a person designated or trained to respond to an emergency. Although we typically think of a police officer, firefighter, or paramedic, there are so many other professions that operate under the umbrella of the definition. I want to be inclusive, because I've learned that there are commonalities among all of these professions when it comes to the effects of stress and trauma.

My challenge, and frankly the challenge of first responders, is breaking through the stoicism and stigma that pervade most of these professions. Traditionally, these cultures encourage first responders to stay quiet about emotional or mental distress. They learn early on that they are expected to accept the inevitability of organizational stress and dysfunction, debilitating stress symptoms, emotional upheaval, sleep disruption and disorders, marriage problems and divorce, and substance use and abuse.

The coping mechanisms that are most often modeled and accepted in these cultures include excessive drinking, the use of prescription drugs, risky behavior, avoidance, and black humor (telling jokes and laughing about the shocking, disturbing, and gruesome things being experienced on the job). Makes sense, doesn't it? If a person isn't allowed to feel and show normal human emotions, at least the laughter provides some relief from the bottled-up pain, grief, sorrow, anger, fear, and despondency.

Meditation and mindfulness are coping mechanisms that can help a person learn to modulate stress and emotion for the purpose of self-regulation. They require stillness and silence, and yes, they require observation and *feeling*. But wait, there's more.

These powerful personal practices can also empower a person to choose *focus* and *intensity* when needed, and de-escalation when desired. Can you imagine this level of self-discipline and relief?

For those of you concerned that you'll lose your edge, please don't worry. I'm not asking you to sit down and meditate in the middle of a crisis. Rather, I'm suggesting that you use these tools between crises and train yourself to harness the power to defuse and de-stress when you need to or want to.

Hypervigilance is a big problem in the first-responder community. Yes, your senses need to be heightened at work, and your ability to focus and react is what makes you an excellent first responder. But you might not need the same level of intensity on every call or with every interaction, especially at home. The problem is, hypervigilance gets locked in, stresses your biological systems, and can hurt the people around you. Same with anger, hostility, aggression, defensiveness, negativity, and apathy.

So, I'm asking first responders to set aside their preconceptions and skepticism and give me a chance—to give meditation and mindfulness a chance. The status quo is not working. Our first responders are stressed and traumatized, and they are dying at alarming rates, sometimes prematurely, due to stress-related health problems, sometimes in line-of-duty deaths, and way too often by their own hand.

What I present, in my classes and in this book, is an introduction to the concept of meditation and mindfulness as healing tools. I am offering a simple, straightforward, logical way for you to dip your big toe into the pool, so to speak. If, when you finish this book, meditation appeals to you on any level, but you are not connecting with my style of instruction, please don't give up! All it takes is a quick search of the internet to find other practices and techniques. I promise, you can find something that works for you.

Also, you should know, I *am* teaching cops to meditate, and they are loving it! In fact, I'm working with first responders from all professions and they are embracing these once new-agey, now mainstream practices with open arms. Well, they embrace them with open arms after begrudgingly sitting in class with their arms crossed in front of them for the first thirty minutes. I love the challenge!

So here we go. Uncross your arms and set those preconceptions aside. I have some things I'd like to share with you, because I really want you to live a long, healthy, happy life. You deserve it.

Part 1

# THE
# WARRIOR

# Chapter 1

# FROM WIDOW TO WARRIOR

"Show me a hero and I'll write you a tragedy."

**—F. Scott Fitzgerald**

My husband dedicated thirty years of his life to a profession that trains warriors for battle but has no context for healing the invisible wounds of warfare. Did the job kill my husband? No. Was it a contributor? Absolutely.

Our first responders are very well trained, but their training does not prepare them for the mental and emotional impacts of the job.

## INVISIBLE WOUNDS

A majority of first responders suffer from symptoms of post-traumatic stress, which is a condition that develops in some people who encounter trauma. Trauma is a deeply distressing or disturbing experience that alters a person's ability to cope.

The average citizen has no idea what first responders see, hear, and endure throughout their careers. They are constantly exposed to and affected by the trauma of others: accidents, disaster, violence, abuse, neglect, victimization, and death. This type of trauma is known as secondary trauma.

First responders regularly encounter scenes and circumstances that most of us could not stomach. The sights, sounds, and smells from these experiences leave imprints on their psyches. Memories and images can continue to harm them after the event is over, and very often these invisible wounds do not heal on their own.

Post-traumatic stress (PTS) and secondary trauma are not visible like a burn, a gunshot wound, or a laceration. They occur on the inside, unseen, but they cause just as much, if not more, pain.

Left untreated, PTS and secondary trauma can be stealthy killers. They quietly ruin health, relationships, families, and lives. They can cause people to withdraw and isolate, or rage and lash out. They create devastation and rob individuals of the most basic human rights: life, love, and joy. However, they are treatable. But in order for treatment to become normalized, the shame and disgrace attached to seeking help must be eliminated.

## Stigma

There has long been a stigma attached to mental health issues in these often stoic emergency-responder professions. If a person is brave (or desperate) enough to speak up about mental and emotional difficulties, they face the possibility of being labeled "weak," "unstable," or "incompetent." Instead of receiving help, they might be demoted—or fired. This ridiculous stigma causes first responders to suffer in silence, forced to pretend they're okay when they're not.

This is what my husband did, for years and years. In order to survive in the law enforcement culture, David felt he had to remain silent about anxiety, depression, and other symptoms he suffered over the years. He was terrified of being deemed incompetent or unsuitable for the job. He worried about being stripped of his badge and gun and being fired without the ability to support his family and collect the pension he had worked so hard to build.

I want to make a point here about mental health and first responders, and I want to address first responders directly.

Getting treatment for mental health does not mean you are mentally ill. I try to always include the word "emotional," when speaking about first responders who need help, because mental and emotional distress go hand in hand when they are caused by a stressful, traumatic profession. I say mental and emotional difficulties, or mental and emotional problems or issues.

I think one of the main reasons you haven't sought or won't seek help is that you don't want people to think you're mentally ill or crazy. First of all, mental illness is not the same as being crazy, and everyone needs to knock it off with that kind of language and thinking. Secondly, mental illness is treatable, is not necessarily permanent, and should never be stigmatized.

So, listen up! You have been mentally and emotionally wounded. This should not cause shame any more than a physical wound would.

If you are struggling mentally and emotionally because of the work you do and the things you've seen, you have been wounded. You are not weak, you are human.

And let me be blunt. If you are resistant to help and treatment because of the stigma, you are sacrificing your life to your job, and that is unacceptable. Some day you will leave this job, one way or another, and when you do, what will your life look like?

How is your mental, emotional, and physical health? What about your personal life, your relationships, and your social life? Are you happy, healthy, and thriving? Or do you operate in some version of survival mode, putting one foot in front of the other in a joyless existence?

I've met a lot of veteran and retired first responders who have been divorced more than once, drink too much, suffer from chronic health problems, and have adult children who won't speak to them. So, if your plan is to give everything to your job and then be happy when you retire, consider this. When you retire, assuming you live that long, all the garbage that you've stuffed down and held in will still be there. It doesn't magically disappear. It rots and festers. And, the day after you retire, the job goes on as if you never existed. Which means the job is just fine, whether you're there or not.

Are you willing to give everything to a job that will not miss a beat when you leave?

And now I want to address leaders and commanders.

It is imperative that you immediately initiate and execute policies to end this stigma. This is a top-down situation that can only be fixed by the people at the top showing real leadership and compassion. Old-fashioned, outdated thinking must be tossed out the window. It's time for the old-guard, "suck it up" leaders to retire and step aside if they are unwilling to embrace empathy and understanding.

If I hear about one more boss saying they don't believe in PTSD (post-traumatic stress disorder), I think I will likely explode. If this is your mindset, it is time for you to hang it up, madam or sir. The world has passed you by and, not only are you standing in the way of progress, but your misinformed and misguided rhetoric and decisions are killing people.

## Ripple Effects

I would be remiss in speaking to first responders and commanders if I didn't address the ripple effects that occur when someone does make the choice to end their own life.

I've heard from people who have considered suicide, and some who have even attempted it, that at the point of choice, they believed everyone in their lives would be better off without them. Somehow, in the midst of feeling like they're drowning in pain, fear, anxiety, depression, and despair, people who are suicidal rationalize that death is the only answer—the only relief. I'm sure there are many different versions of this, but as I understand it, it goes something like this: *I am a mess, I am so tired of feeling like this, nothing helps, I have become a burden to my friends and family, and everyone will be better off with me gone. They'll all be fine eventually and my suffering will end. This is just for the best.*

While this is hard for most of us to understand, I believe some people reach a point where they have lost all memory of what it's like to feel okay, and they are so exhausted from suffering that they convince themselves death is their only path to peace and freedom.

If you have considered or are considering suicide, I'd like share with you some of the ripple effects that occurred and continue because of my husband's choice to end his life. The truth is, every person who knew David was negatively impacted in some way. Nobody is better off without him. Not one of us.

David has parents and two sisters who miss him. He has children and stepchildren who miss him and will forever carry heaviness, regret, and pain regarding his choice. He has friends who were shocked, stunned, saddened, and confused by this tragedy.

He had a nephew named Nico, with whom he was especially close. David taught Nico how to fish and use tools. They bonded over "guy stuff," bad jokes, dumb movies, and *Just Dance* on the Wii, which was the most hilarious thing you've ever seen.

Nico struggled with some emotional difficulties in adolescence, and Uncle David was someone he could always talk to. When he found out his uncle had killed himself, he was devastated. We worried about Nico a lot in the days, weeks, and months following David's funeral. Nico made the trip from St. Louis to Kansas City several times in those days to spend time with us. I think being

The Mindfulness for Warriors Handbook

in his uncle's home was comforting somehow. Nico and I were close, and he was close with my kids, especially my son.

On an early Sunday morning in June of 2015, after Nico had spent the night at my house, I talked to him over coffee. I told him I knew he missed his uncle, and that I understood he had been experiencing a rough patch in life. I assured him that I would always be there for him and that he was welcome at our house any time. And then I mustered the courage to say what I *really* wanted to say, which was, "I need to know you're never going to consider killing yourself. I know life gets hard, but you have so many people who love you and this family cannot take another tragedy."

Nico looked me right in the eye and said, "I've seen how much David's death has hurt everyone and I would never consider doing that to my family." I was so relieved.

On July 2, 2015, seven months after David ended his own life with a self-inflicted gunshot wound to the head, Nicholas "Nico" Hundelt did the exact same thing. He was twenty years old.

Also on that day, David's best friend in the whole world, his sister, Julie, had to face the devastating reality that she had lost her brother and closest friend, as well as her youngest child, in the span of less than a year.

The ripples continue.

Nico has a mom and a dad who miss him terribly and will never stop grieving. He has two brothers who loved him so much and have to face each day knowing their little brother is gone forever. He had a girlfriend when he died. He had more friends than you could count, and at least a couple of them have since experienced their own darkness, depression, and even suicidal ideation.

Did you know that suicide can be contagious? There is something called "suicide contagion." It's a phenomenon that occurs in families and peer groups. Basically, exposure to suicide has been shown to increase one's potential to consider suicide.

After Nico's death, the entire family went into a tailspin of emotional and mental anguish and paranoid vigilance. Some family members struggled more than others, and we found ourselves terrified that whoever was not doing well at any given time would be the next one to kill themselves. And I'd be lying if I told you we've stopped worrying about that.

Every one of us has indelible and unshakeable memories of how and when we found out about each of these deaths, and now many of us are triggered by the simplest things, like late-night phone calls, calls from a family member at an unusual time, or a knock at the door. We were each shocked, stunned, and devastated by the deaths of these men we loved so much.

So, if you are someone who is considering suicide, know this. If you choose suicide, and you have children, you have just modeled for them that suicide is an option when life gets hard. When those children encounter dark times in life, and they are searching for answers, help, and relief, they are much more likely to consider suicide. Is that the legacy you want to leave behind? And it's not just your kids you might unwittingly be giving permission. Friends, family members, and colleagues might also be more likely to follow suit.

Suicide does not end suffering. It simply passes suffering on to others.

# Silent Suffering

David was a police officer for eight years, from age twenty-one to twenty-nine, and then he joined a federal agency and worked as a Special Agent and a SAC (Special Agent in Charge) for twenty-two years. I believe most of his buried trauma occurred during the eight years he was on patrol. In my travels with the PauseFirst Project, I've met many people who worked with David over the years. They have all been generous in their praise of his police work and investigative skills.

My husband was *good* at his job, but he was not *built* for the job. Since his death, I have learned that nobody is, not really. Humans are not built to endure and withstand years and years of intense stress, trauma, death, and devastation. Yes, there are people who can do the work and do it well, but nobody goes unscathed. David was a sweet, sensitive, emotional man at his core. The dysfunction, death, and violence he witnessed as a police officer affected him deeply and subsequently impacted his entire life.

In a later segment in this book, titled "His Buried Trauma," I will talk more about what David endured during his eight years as a patrolman. Those early years caused indelible pain and trauma that I believe changed the trajectory of my husband's life.

In my opinion, had David been able to seek assistance for the mental and emotional fallout from the early days on the job, he would have been a more effective law enforcement officer and investigator—and he was pretty damn good as it was. He also could have enjoyed a more peaceful personal life, and he might still be here.

Instead, he struggled and suffered off and on for the entire thirty years, and his suffering caused pain for the people he loved. With knowledge of the stigma surrounding mental and emotional problems in law enforcement so deeply buried in his psyche, instead of seeking help, David became engulfed in a tsunami of trauma symptoms, and ultimately decided death was the only way to escape the pain.

It did not have to be this way, and it doesn't have to end like this for one other first responder.

If any of this resonates with you, if you are a first responder who has suffered similarly, please know there is hope. There is help available. You can heal. You can learn skills and tools to build your resilience and survive, no matter how bad things are.

If you are someone who loves a first responder, and you suspect your loved one is struggling like David did, please know there are first-responder-specific programs and facilities that can help. That is the one piece we were missing near the end of David's life. We did not know that type of help was available. We tried the normal psychiatric route, but that was never going to help my husband because there was no way he was letting his guard down in that environment.

Later in the book, I will offer stories of first responders from all backgrounds: military, law enforcement, fire service, EMS, and dispatch, who at some point in their career found themselves struggling or suffering with post-traumatic stress symptoms, trauma, anxiety, depression, nightmares, recurring memories and images, and even suicidal ideation. They will tell us where they've been, what they experienced, and how it affected them, their families and their lives. Then they will share how they found the courage to step onto a healing path, which tools worked for them, and what they are doing to maintain their well-being.

Maybe you will see yourself in one of these people. Perhaps their story is your story.

If so, my hope is that hearing from these brave and vulnerable souls will create a spark in you and inspire you to take that first step toward wellness and wholeness. Reach out, talk to someone, attend a peer support meeting, or make your first counseling appointment. Learn what helped these people, and maybe try something they tried. But please know that you are not alone. Others have struggled in the same way you are, but they've survived and are thriving, and you can too.

We must put an end to silent suffering. We are losing too many first responders to suicide and premature death due to health problems. First responders deserve a long, full, peaceful, happy, healthy life. They deserve to have connected relationships and a culture and community that supports them.

## My Initiation

Becoming a widow was my initiation as a warrior. I am fighting for first responders and their families. There is a massive nationwide movement to bring healing to our first responders, and I have joined this cause. I'm standing shoulder-to-shoulder with an army of compassionate, caring people who will stop at nothing to help, save, and rescue the brave and important people who have dedicated their lives to helping, saving, and rescuing others. Each of us contributes something unique to the fight, but all of us are united in the commitment to bring sweeping change to this dire situation.

This is not a moment; it's a movement. It's not a wellness fad that will fade away like a trendy diet or the latest health guru. This is a new way of being for first responders and it *will* prevail and sustain.

My small part in this movement is to offer two powerful personal practices to first responders and their families and loved ones. The practices are meditation and mindfulness. These tools help turn one's attention inward, to the self. They can help a person manage stress, regulate emotions, and improve overall health.

Beyond teaching meditation and mindfulness, I am encouraging first responders to seek professional help and step onto a healing path that can change the trajectory of their lives and the lives of everyone they love.

There are many, many other people, other warriors, involved in this movement who are offering myriad tools, therapies, retreats, modalities, education, facilities, books, counseling, peer groups, training, and other forms of support. Together, we *will* make a difference.

If you are a first responder, please join the movement to help and heal, starting with yourself. Up until now, you have *been* the help. Now, maybe you *need* a little help. Please don't allow your stoicism, shame, embarrassment, or pride to keep you from seeking the help and support you need and deserve.

# Chapter 2

# WHAT IS A WARRIOR?

"Be kind, for everyone you meet is fighting a hard battle."

**—Plato**

Here is the most basic, historical definition of a warrior: a person who fights in a battle or war.

Here's my definition: a warrior is anyone who stands ready to serve, protect, and defend a person, place, thing, or cause, and will fight and sacrifice for the betterment of others and for the greater good.

My husband David was a warrior. He was a protector, and a guardian of justice. He had this way of making people feel safe. Once, in marriage counseling, our therapist said, "If the ship is going down, stand next to David and you will survive." That about sums it up. That's who David was at his core.

David was a good man, and he was a good cop, by all accounts. In the year of his death, he received two prominent awards, the State of Missouri Guardian of Justice Award and an MOCIC (Mid-States Organized Crime Information Center) award. In the 1990s, while working as a federal agent, David headed up a two-year-long investigation which led to the arrest and conviction of a crime ring, including a brutal killer who was featured on the TV show *America's Most Wanted*. And he had many other career successes and accolades.

Recently, I was speaking at a law enforcement conference, and I saw a man making a beeline toward me from across the room. As he approached, I thought his eyes looked teary. He stretched out his hand and said, "I worked with your husband many years ago. I hadn't heard that he had passed, I'm so sorry."

I thanked him and we chatted a little. His comments about David echoed what many others have said to me over the years. "Your husband was a really good cop," he said. "If shit was going down, you wanted David there with you."

I always say David was this great combination of a silly, funny, goofy guy who you probably wouldn't want to encounter in a dark alley. He was charming and harmless, until he or someone he felt responsible for was threatened, and then watch out. He could switch to warrior mode in a split second.

The problem is, warring takes a toll on the warrior, and our western society is not good about taking care of these brave and noble individuals.

I've heard that, in ancient times, indigenous people went to great lengths to care for their warriors. When warriors returned home from battle, they were welcomed, honored, and praised. They were given time to reflect and rest and heal. They were tended to and held in high regard. This makes sense to me, considering they put their lives on the line ensuring that others' lives were protected.

## The Gladiator

I have a vivid memory of watching the movie *Gladiator,* starring Russell Crowe, with my husband one night. It was a movie David would watch over and over. I now understand why he was drawn to that story. He identified with the main character. Not in a dreamy, wishful way. He literally possessed the traits of the gladiator, but he would never have admitted that, because he was also humble.

The movie is about a principled man and revered Roman general who seeks revenge against a corrupt emperor who ordered the murder of the general's family, captured and enslaved him, and forced him to fight in the gladiator arena.

During a particularly brutal fight scene, I said something to my husband like, "I hate watching this violent stuff. I hate war. I hate fighting. It's just not my thing."

David paused the movie, looked at me and replied, "Well, you better be glad there are people willing to get into the arena and fight." I said, "I know. You're right. And I am grateful for that."

He was absolutely right, and he wasn't just referring to the movie, or the gladiator arena. My off-the-cuff comment triggered something in him about people who abhor violence and have dreams of a peaceful world. I realize, looking back, that in his role as a law enforcement officer, David did not seek out conflict or violence, it was thrust upon him.

Just a few weeks after David died, I watched *Gladiator* by myself. I probably cried more watching that movie than I cried at David's funeral. My husband embodied all the qualities of Maximus Decimus Meridius, Commander of the Armies of the North, General of the Felix Legions, and loyal servant to the true Emperor, Marcus Aurelius.

David was principled, brave, determined, loyal, and protective, especially if he loved you. He understood that doing a job well meant sacrifice. He took pride in everything he did. You could count on him. You felt safe with him.

He identified with that movie because he *was* a gladiator. He didn't want to fight, but if you threw him into the arena, he would survive. Maximus quickly became a leader to the other slaves in the arena and used his instincts and ability, not only to save himself, but to keep the other slaves alive as well. That was how David lived his life—with a high degree of honor and sense of responsibility.

A warrior is a gladiator, a fighter, a protector, and a hero. Their innate instinct to survive and save others far surpasses what the rest of us possess.

## Keep Fighting

If your life or work involves helping, saving, and rescuing others in any capacity, large or small, you are a warrior. If you are someone who stands ready to serve, protect, and defend a person, place, thing, or cause, and will fight and sacrifice for the betterment of others and for the greater good, you are a warrior.

You are a warrior. I am the wife of a warrior, now a widow and a warrior myself. We've been thrown into the arena, and we need to keep fighting, all of us. For ourselves, our well-being, and our families, for others, and for the greater good.

# Chapter 3

# DEATH NOTIFICATION

The Saturday after Thanksgiving in 2014 was unseasonably warm in Kansas City.

My thirteen-year-old daughter and I took advantage of the nice weather and hung some Christmas lights on our front porch, then I drove her to a friend's house for a sleepover. When I got back home, I started making dinner.

As I stirred a pot on my stove, I heard a knock. I walked toward the front door, and as I got closer, I could see a uniformed officer standing on my porch.

A feeling I cannot put into words flooded my entire system, and as I type, the feeling returns.

I opened the door, and the officer began to speak. It's impossible to explain the shock and paralyzing emotion that engulfed me in the next few seconds. My husband had been found in his truck, in the back of our neighborhood, with a self-inflicted gunshot wound to his head. He was gone.

The next few hours, days, weeks, and months are a blurry mess in my memory. My husband chose a permanent solution to a temporary problem, and in the process created untold waves of pain and trauma.

Like everyone else who's ever grieved, I swirled around in a vortex of sadness, anger, fear, regret, resentment, nostalgia, love, longing, confusion, and finally, acceptance (after a long, long time).

The distance, time, and space between me and that life-altering day in 2014 eventually gave rise to something new. I began to think about that incident in a new way, from a different perspective. It started with something I remembered the police officer saying in my doorway. He mentioned that an off-duty firefighter was the one who heard the shot, found my husband, and called 911. At the time, I think I had a fleeting sense of relief that it was a first responder and not a neighborhood kid who found him.

Next, my mind began to wander from person to person who might have been involved in that horrific call that day. Besides the caller, there would have been a dispatcher. What a terrible call to receive. Then, there would have been all of the others who were dispatched to the scene and had to see it, work it, keep citizens away, and participate in the cleanup. And, finally, the coroner.

It was extremely difficult for me to allow myself to picture the scene at all, let alone picturing it in such vivid detail. But there was something inside me trying to get my attention. It was nudging me toward the proper empathy and compassion for, not only the individuals who had to work the scene of a suicide that day, but *all* of the people who do this kind of work every day.

I realized it must have been awful for the officer who came to my house, and the detective who accompanied him and had to give me all the pertinent information in a matter-of-fact way while he watched me melting and dissolving into a puddle of grief right before his eyes.

Oh my God. My husband had done this work. Dots started connecting in my head and heart.

Prior to becoming a federal investigator, David was a police officer for eight years. He went on horrific calls and processed gruesome crime scenes. He knocked on doors and told mothers their child had died. He saw death and violence, devastation and destruction, and he witnessed things so heinous he wouldn't speak of them.

This realization started slowly and gained momentum steadily. The more I thought about it, the more shocked I was that this had never occurred to me before. Of course, police work had contributed to my husband's overall mental and emotional health issues. Of course, he carried invisible wounds and trauma that impacted his worldview and affected every aspect of his well-being. Of course. Of course. They all do.

All first responders have invisible wounds. They see, hear, and endure things that most of us can't even imagine. They carry a weight that would be unbearable for the average citizen, and because of this, they are dying younger and, in some cases, choosing to end their own lives.

So, if there's something I can do to help other first responders manage their stress and find a bit of relief from this taxing and traumatic way of life, I want to do it. I have to do it. As a tribute to my husband and a thank-you to these great people, I must do what I can to help.

## Part 2

# THE WEIGHT

# Chapter 4

# HIS BURIED TRAUMA

### The Effects of Accumulated Stress and Trauma

Since David's suicide, I've learned a lot about trauma and secondary trauma, and how they can permeate and affect every aspect of a person's life. My husband carried a tremendous amount of trauma that had roots in his early years, grew exponentially throughout his police career, and affected all areas of his life.

## THE IMPACTS OF TRAUMA

Trauma occurs when a person experiences or witnesses abuse, victimization, neglect, loss, violence, and disasters. The term "secondary trauma" refers to exposure to the trauma of others. Unfortunately, the majority of first responders experience some kind of trauma during their career, and it can be toxic to them mentally and emotionally. To make things worse, many first responders are carrying around trauma they incurred prior to embarking on their career.

This is certainly true in David's case, and I want to share with you a couple of experiences he had early on that I believe initiated, or at least contributed to, his lifelong struggle with anxiety and depression.

### Age Sixteen

When David was only sixteen years old, he and three friends were in a car on a country road. David was seated in the back seat, behind the passenger. The driver lost control of the car and started to veer off the road. There was a downed telephone pole on the side of the road. David saw it and ducked as the pole crashed through the windshield, decapitating his friend sitting in front of him. David was not injured.

As David recounted this story, what struck me was the fact that the three surviving boys received no counseling of any kind. Of course, this would have been around 1980, a time in which counseling and therapy were not ubiquitous, as they are now. However, I suspect this traumatizing experience did more damage to David emotionally and psychologically than anyone knew. He definitely had survivor's guilt, often wondering why *he* was able to avoid the pole, but his friend wasn't.

### Age Twenty-One

In my husband's first year of policing, when he was only twenty-one years old, he was involved in a shootout that began with him being shot at, and which resulted in his killing the shooter. Afterwards, he was called in to the police station, where his badge and gun were taken away and he was sent home.

David spent the next several days in an apartment alone, afraid, and isolated, not knowing what was going to happen to him. Then he got a call telling him that the incident had been ruled "suicide by police," and he had been cleared. They told him to report for roll call the next day. When he returned, he was given his badge and gun, went to roll call, and climbed back into a patrol car. And that was that. Back to work. No counseling, no conversation, no debrief, and no support of any kind.

When I think of all of the trauma this incident caused, it makes my heart heavy. For starters, he was only twenty-one. I can't imagine the trauma of being shot at, fearing for your life, and then ultimately taking someone else's life. I know this incident haunted him because, whenever he talked about it, which was rare, he would become extremely emotional. He could never reconcile, in his head and heart, taking the life of another human being. And he lived with that guilt until the day he died.

## The Cost of Untreated Trauma

If nothing else upsetting had ever occurred in David's life, these two incidents alone would be enough to cause distress. But that wasn't the case. David encountered a tremendous amount of stress and trauma in his lifetime, and much of it was concentrated in the eight years he served as a police officer. As a federal agent for the final twenty-two years of his career, he worked some difficult cases and encountered challenges, but nothing like those eight years in a patrol car. Those years were brutal.

Yet he never sought, nor did he receive, proper treatment.

Throughout David's career, the untreated and unprocessed trauma caused him to experience recurring symptoms, which he was intermittently able to numb—typically with alcohol. He battled with anxiety and depression off and on, and he suffered from recurring dreams and nightmares. In his dreams, there were three consistent themes: he was in a police station, he felt a sense of being lost or in the wrong place, and he often needed to discharge his weapon but could not. He would even wake up with a sore hand from squeezing it tightly and repeatedly in his sleep.

Over time, accumulated stress and trauma grew so overwhelming and so powerful that it infiltrated David's personality, turning an otherwise great guy into an angry, paranoid, cynical character, or an emotional wreck who could not stop crying. These stress-induced symptoms ultimately left my husband unable to cope with change, uncertainty, or the most basic daily challenges.

As he approached retirement, I believe all the unprocessed pain, fear, anxiety, and depression that he had contained over the years began creeping up and oozing into every crack and crevice, flooding and engulfing him mercilessly. He began taking an antidepressant. That didn't help. He added an anti-anxiety drug. That didn't help. He drank. That didn't help. He kept himself busy. That didn't help—and *that* had always helped.

## THE DARK SIDE OF THE LIGHT OF MY LIFE

It has taken me a long time to summon the courage to speak honestly about my husband, his issues, and our struggles. David was a very proud and private man, so telling his secrets feels like a betrayal of sorts.

I don't want to let strangers into the dark corners of our life together. I'd much rather talk about the good times, and there were plenty of those. Anyone who knew us knew that we loved each other deeply and shared an intimate friendship that I may never know again. But toward the end of his life, when he was unraveling, that changed, and he turned on me.

My sweet, loving husband became someone I hardly recognized and could rarely reason with. He vacillated between despair, anger, bouts of crying, and hostility. He said and did things that were out of character and extremely hurtful, and he made some choices he would never have made in his right mind.

The last few months of his life were like the scariest roller coaster you can imagine, with hairpin turns, inversions, barrel rolls, negative Gs, no brakes, and no seat belts. The man I had known to be as solid as a rock was up and down and all over the place, unpredictable and inconsistent in every way.

What I now know, having interacted with a lot of first responders and their spouses, is that a high percentage of spouses experience the roller coaster at some point in their relationship, if not throughout. It's terrifying to be on the receiving end of that kind of whiplash, especially if you are trying to keep a marriage and family together.

The truth is, throughout our marriage, there was a dark side to David that cast a shadow on our otherwise sunny life—like a murky figure lurking in the background. When he got emotionally triggered by anger or felt threatened in any way, this dark figure would step out of the shadows and take over. This happened rarely, but when it did, it was intense.

That dark guy was never violent toward me, but he was angry and hateful and completely out of control. After each "episode" had subsided, David was embarrassed, ashamed, and apologetic.

And, even though these episodes were awful, I felt so sorry for my husband because it was clear he was full of pain. I believe this dark alter ego developed as a result of years of unresolved trauma and suffering.

In the last days, there was very little left of the David I had known and loved. His eyes were vacant, and his personality was totally altered. On the day he died, however, he left me with a gift. As we were passing each other in our bedroom, he reached out and stopped me. He stood in front of me, placed his hands on my shoulders, stared right into my eyes, and said, "I love you."

I replied with an exasperated, "I love you too, David." But then I looked into his eyes, and I saw something I hadn't seen for months. Clarity. He did not let go of me as he went on. "I love you, honey. I really love you. I need you to know that I love you." "I love you, too," I replied again, and I put my arms around him. We hugged for a long time in silence. That was the first lucidity I had witnessed in a long time, and our last embrace.

## My Message to Spouses

In my early days of teaching first responders, a firefighter gave me one of the best gifts ever. After class, he caught me in the hall, and we had a brief, private chat. He thanked me for my work and extended his condolences for the loss of my husband. Then he said something important.

He told me very kindly that he detected a lack of confidence in my delivery and referred back to some comments I had made like, "Now, I know I'm not a first responder and can never really understand what you've experienced."

Then he looked at me and said, "You are a first responder. You were married to one of us, and that makes you one of us." He went on to say, "This is what I tell my wife, and I mean it. It is not easy being married to someone who does this work, and I know sometimes you guys take the brunt of the stress. So," he said, "don't ever diminish yourself. You are one of us."

That was a real confidence-booster and a bit of validation I didn't even realize I needed. Most first responders avoid telling their spouses about the horrific things they see at work as a way to shield and protect them. But ironically, holding these stories in causes the emotional damage to accumulate. A human being can only hold a certain amount of stress, anger, trauma, sadness, fear, and depression before the unbearable pressure demands release. Unfortunately, they usually release it on the people closest to them, and this is most often their spouse, and sometimes their children.

If you're married to a first responder who is struggling, you are most likely not doing well yourself, and you probably have no idea what to do. It is scary to see the person you love, or once loved, unravel, withdraw, and rage. One of the hardest parts of a relationship like this is the helplessness we feel that we can't fix, save, or rescue them.

I'm not qualified to guide or counsel anyone, but I will encourage you to reach out for the help that is available until you find the right fit. Seek out first-responder-specific programs and trauma-informed-care therapists. Take care of yourself and your children, and if there is domestic violence involved, take immediate steps to get and keep everyone safe, no matter what it takes.

Whatever you do, please don't continue to live in pain and dysfunction. First responders aren't the only ones who sometimes suffer in silence; spouses are susceptible to all the same issues. If you are suffering, you can be guaranteed your children are suffering also. Please reach out, find a peer support group, talk to other spouses, try counseling—*anything* that might help to heal the situation.

## THE VULNERABILITY PARADOX

I observed and endured a lot of dysfunction as a result of my husband's unresolved trauma. This is extremely difficult for me to admit because I feel vulnerable exposing the underbelly of my imperfect private life. I guess I'm afraid of being judged.

As I identify this feeling of vulnerability within myself, I realize this is the very fear that gripped my husband and kept him from seeking the help he needed. I have deep compassion for this man who, in order to survive and thrive in the law enforcement culture, felt he could not afford to be vulnerable.

That's the tangled web, isn't it? First responders are hurting or scared, but they want people to think they're okay. If they are honest about their struggles, if they say they need help, others might think they are weak or broken or crazy. Not to mention the fact that they could face demotion or dismissal from their jobs. So they stay quiet. And they suffer.

The deeper I get into my work with first responders, the more I realize how important it is for me to let my guard down and speak the truth about my husband's problems and our mostly awesome, but sometimes awful, life together. There are too many people suffering in silence and *way* too many people dying. I hope that David's story—our story—will shine a light on this reality so others won't have to endure the same pain and tragedy.

## The Unraveling

In the year leading up to my husband's death, his mental health became increasingly worse. His decision to retire after thirty years triggered a surge of anxiety and, although he had spent two years carefully crafting a new business venture with a partner, David was terrified of the uncertainty of civilian life and wallowed in thoughts about worst-case scenarios.

In hindsight, there were all kinds of warning signs during that year. David's anxiety intensified and the "episodes," which were almost always alcohol-induced, became more frequent. The dark guy surfaced more often and brought with him fear, worry, angst, paranoia, and irrational behavior.

David's last day at work was Friday, September 5, 2014. On Saturday, we had his retirement party. On Sunday, he had a full-blown anxiety attack, and by the following week his anxiety sent him to the emergency room. This kicked off two months of intense inpatient and outpatient treatment, and the slew of prescription medications did not help. In fact, they made things worse.

He barely made it through Thanksgiving dinner because the anxiety was so intense that he could not sit still, or focus, or even carry on a normal conversation. Two days later, David killed himself.

# Hindsight

I wish I had known then what I know now about the impacts of trauma and the specialized help that's available. My biggest regret is that I was not aware of any first-responder-specific treatment programs. Many of them have sprung up in the years since David's death, and the ones that existed just never showed up on my radar. I searched, and researched, but I didn't have the awareness I do today, so I wasn't looking in the right places.

David was admitted to psychiatric care via the emergency room and participated in both inpatient and outpatient programs. He did not feel like this was the right care for him. I remember him saying, "I'm sitting in a circle with drug addicts talking about their addictions. This is not helping me. This is not what I need."

Now that I'm aware of first-responder-specific facilities and treatment programs, and the trauma-informed care approach, I agree. He was absolutely right. The care he received was not the care he needed.

## Chapter 5

# DARKNESS TO LIGHT

**First Responders Share Stories of Difficult
Times and How They Are Healing**

## THE POWER OF STORYTELLING

I've been working exclusively with first responders since 2017,
and I've noticed some patterns and commonalities that I feel
are important to note. In each talk I deliver and every class I
teach, certain attendees approach me to chat during breaks or
after the conclusion of my presentation.

A high percentage of people who want to talk to me are on the
older side, typically over the age of forty. They are veterans in
their field. They've been there and done that, and something
about my story causes something in them to stir. Some of them
see themselves in David's story. Others are beginning to think
about retirement and are feeling the fear, worry, and anxiety
creep in. Still others simply identify me as a safe person to

whom they can tell their tale. So I listen with my ears and my heart, because I am honored that they trust me with their story.

A few months ago, when I was on the road, I was conducting an in-service training for a large group of primarily law enforcement officers. During the class, I noticed several times that a small group of people, sitting together near the back of the room, weren't taking the training seriously. They looked to be about twenty-five to thirty in age, and they chatted a lot among themselves and were basically just screwing around.

Conversely, there were several individuals in the front rows who seemed to be taking the class very seriously. They were older—I would guess in the forty-five-to-sixty-five age range. A couple of times during my presentation, especially when I was talking about David and the impact of accumulated stress, I noticed a few of them were teary-eyed. As I observed this and made mental notes about the glaringly different response coming from the goofballs in the back, I had an *aha* moment.

It occurred to me that the younger ones weren't as engaged because they didn't think they needed this stress-reduction stuff. They're young, they've only been on the job for a couple of years, and they still feel invincible. They haven't clocked the hours, haven't logged the miles. Their resilience hasn't been depleted.

But the veteran people, the cops with a lot of years under their belts, they were listening. They were leaning in and taking notes. They saw themselves in David's story when I spoke of the trauma he had endured and how he carried it, unprocessed and unhealed, for decades. I suspect that somewhere deep inside they know that they too will be vulnerable to mental and

The Mindfulness for Warriors Handbook

emotional unraveling at retirement if they don't do something to lessen the psychological burdens they carry.

Even if the young people don't think they need classes and stress-reduction tools now, I know I'm planting seeds. I know that someday the goofballs in the back will be the veterans in the front. Hopefully, as they navigate their careers, the seeds will take root, and when they begin to feel the weight of the job, they will remember my class and David's story and, instead of allowing things to pile up, they will reach out for help or seek a healing path.

My experience with the young goofballs and the teary veterans served as a reminder that David's story is important and needs to be told. In fact, I believe that the sharing of stories in an honest and vulnerable way will be the single most important catalyst for change. That's why I wanted to write this book and share the stories of some of the brave and vulnerable first responders I've met through my work.

These people have worked in service to community and country. They have seen, heard, witnessed, and endured things that most of us can't even imagine. They carry burdens and images and memories that they can't fully unload, can't completely erase.

I have the utmost respect for this group of people, and I consider them to be the bravest of the brave, because they have chosen to tell their stories. It takes grit and guts to be honest, to put oneself out there and admit to frailties and vulnerabilities. The level of courage it takes to speak up in a profession that prides itself on silence and stoicism is commendable.

Let's discuss how their strength and willingness toward vulnerability is inspiring others and changing cultures.

I've noticed that, when one person is courageous enough to speak the truth about their struggles and pain, they create an opening for the next person to speak up. It's like the courage is contagious. Suddenly, someone else who has kept their suffering bottled up feels safe enough to share *their* experiences and feelings, because they no longer feel alone. This causes a chain reaction of sharing, caring, support, and community that serves to heal the invisible wounds.

When one person steps forward and says, "I'm hurting," it paves the way for others to step forward as well. People need to be seen, valued, and validated. I believe this is human nature, not a flaw or a weakness. When courageous people share what has happened to them and how it is affecting them, others feel safe to say they are hurting too. If everyone remains silent, then everyone thinks everyone else is doing okay but them. This deepens the feelings of shame and the fear that they will be seen as weak, and this nonsense is killing people.

Verbally sharing lived experience of trauma can be cathartic and healing for both the speaker and the listener.

So, without further ado, let's meet the first responders.

I sat down with some veteran first responders and asked them the following five questions:

1. What is your background?
2. Can you share a little about some of the difficult experiences you've endured?

The Mindfulness for Warriors Handbook

3. Was there a turning point?

4. Which tools have you found most useful on your journey?

5. What needs to change in these cultures to support well-being?

Sometimes we stuck to the script, other times our conversations veered off course, but in every single instance, the answers were profound.

Here's what they had to say.

# • JUSTIN •

**Military**

United States Army Infantryman, 25th ID, 1st,
SBCT (Stryker Brigade Combat Team)

One tour in support of Operation
Iraqi Freedom 2004–2005

I got connected with Justin because of my work with the PauseFirst Project and his work with The Battle Within (a five-day retreat in nature for veterans and first responders). Our first meeting was in a coffee shop in early 2019. I learned all about The Battle Within, how the organization came to be, and how Justin became involved. I loved everything I heard.

Justin is smart and articulate and has a personality that puts you at ease. I knew right off the bat he was someone I would love to work with, so I was thrilled when he reached out a few months later and invited me to lead mindfulness and meditation sessions at The Battle Within retreats. I am enjoying that work immensely, and I get to spend time with some pretty awesome people when I'm there.

I sat down with Justin in my living room and asked him about his time in Iraq. I wasn't prepared for what he was about to share. The realities of war are shocking, and Justin was only twenty years old when he deployed.

## Difficult Experiences

In Tal Afar, Iraq, Justin's company was charged with guarding the last standing police station in the area. During this time, two of the Iraqi police officers were captured, tortured, killed, and left out on the street. The other cops were, understandably, extremely upset by this. The US soldiers pleaded with the men to wait for EOD (Explosive Ordnance Disposal) to come clear the bodies, because insurgents would often hide explosives on dead bodies. The police officers refused to listen. Two of them went to retrieve the bodies and explosives embedded within the bodies killed them both.

After this incident, the other police officers were in the police station, drinking heavily. All of them were armed, which was clearly not a good situation, plus there was a lot of unspoken tension between the police and the infantrymen. At some point, one of the police officers left, unbeknownst to the US soldiers charged with defending them.

The officer walked unnoticed into the marketplace and opened fire on civilians. Luckily, the US soldiers were able to stop the man and arrest him.

Later that day, Justin's team went to the local hospital for some kind of meeting. As he walked down the hall, he noticed a young girl on a gurney in the hallway by herself. She had been injured in the marketplace shooting. She was gray. He assumed she was dead.

At this point in our conversation, Justin provided a sidebar. He told me that, by this time in his tour, he was closed-off emotionally. He said, in order to survive over there, you pretty much had to turn off your feelings and emotions.

As he walked by the girl on the gurney, he noticed that her chest was moving just a bit. She was still alive, but just barely. He kept walking. And later he learned that the girl had died.

As a matter of survival in a war zone, soldiers are forced to shut off their emotions and stay focused on the business at hand. I got the impression talking to Justin that the decision to keep walking as he passed the dying girl wasn't a conscious one. It was the order of the day: stay sharp, keep going, take care of your own, and survive.

While he was deployed in Iraq, Justin's vehicle was impacted by twenty-two separate incidents of IEDs (improvised explosive devices), a car bomb, and a suicide car bomb. He suffered a TBI (traumatic brain injury) along with other non-life-threatening injuries.

He was once trapped in an alley, with one other soldier and an Iraqi interpreter, when an Iraqi soldier opened fire. The three were pinned down, exchanging gunfire, and a bullet grazed Justin's temple. As the RTO (radiotelephone operator), Justin was able to call for reinforcements to gain fire superiority, and all three made it out alive. Later, a doctor told Justin that, had the bullet struck a half-inch over, he would have been dead.

Justin was awarded two Purple Hearts.

He lost people in his company while fighting in Iraq, and has since lost several more to suicide.

## Turning Point

It wasn't until about ten years after returning home that Justin realized something was wrong. During an extremely difficult time in which his stepdaughter was struggling with depression and suicidal ideation, Justin noticed that experiences and memories from Iraq began to surface.

His stepdaughter was in and out of treatment facilities at that time. Spending time in a hospital setting and seeing his stepdaughter on a hospital bed triggered images and memories of the young girl on the gurney in that hospital in Tal Afar. He couldn't stop thinking about her. He wondered if anyone was with her when she died. He wished he had stopped to help her. He second-guessed their decision to arrest the shooter and wondered, if had they had killed him instead, might the girl still be alive?

These are the kinds of thoughts, memories, and images that haunt military veterans. No human being is built to witness death, destruction, and atrocities en masse and keep going. These experiences cause trauma that gets locked into the mind, heart, and even the body.

Justin says his wife and mother had noticed changes in him when he returned from Iraq, despite his own assessment that he was doing fine. Ten years later, as the signs of post-traumatic stress began to surface during his stepdaughter's crisis, Justin's wife demanded that he get some help. And that was the beginning of his healing journey.

He started with a five-day retreat for military veterans. This was the first time he realized, or at least the first time he admitted, that he might have PTSD.

Next, Justin tried therapy, where he experienced EMDR (eye movement desensitization and reprocessing), a technique used to relieve psychological stress. He says EMDR was effective and helped him process the thoughts and emotions that haunted him around the girl on the hospital gurney.

Next, he attended another five-day retreat. This one was for military veterans and first responders. He found the second retreat to be more effective, primarily because the first one had presented brief introductions to some healing modalities like yoga and meditation, but the second one offered a more immersive experience, by integrating these new practices into each day. That, he says, enabled him to feel the benefits and improvements by the time he left.

This retreat also provided Justin with one of the most important elements of his healing process: community.

After returning home from Iraq, Justin felt a deep void and experienced an unexpected grieving period, realizing he would never have the depth of connection, solidarity, and community he had experienced in the Army. He missed his military family.

The retreat filled that void by bringing together ten men with similar backgrounds who bonded, shared, and healed together over the course of the week. Justin left that retreat knowing *this* was his new community. Their connection, he says, was genuine and authentic, and he knew it would endure. When he left the retreat, he knew he could reach out to any member of this group, or any alumnus or mentor of the program, at any time, and he would be supported. The group has stayed connected and continues to support the healing journey of each individual.

## Tools

### Mindfulness, Community, EMDR Therapy

According to Justin, the tools he has found most helpful on his healing journey are mindfulness, community, and EMDR therapy.

## What Needs to Change

Justin ticked off a list of changes he believes would improve military and veteran wellness and curtail the epidemic of suicide.

Developing resiliency programs prior to deployment.

- Reducing stigma through peer support programs.

- Post-enlistment, having a better handoff to veteran community and VSOs (veterans service organizations) so there isn't a lapse in community that leads to isolation, depression, and suicide.

Justin currently serves as Executive Director of The Battle Within (thebattlewithin.org), a five-day healing journey in nature for veterans and first responders, located in Kansas City, Missouri.

# • BRENDA •

### Law Enforcement

Twenty-eight years

Colonel, retired as an undersheriff
in charge of jail operations;

Spent the majority of her career in
patrol and investigations

Brenda and I sat down at my kitchen table and visited over lunch. She seems to be doing very well, and I wanted to know how she managed to retire so healthfully after almost thirty years on the job.

After lunch, we moved to my couch and she started to open up about her years in law enforcement. She said, as she approached retirement, she realized she had been through a lot, so she decided to try a little therapy, just to make sure everything was okay. She believes that decision played a huge role in her healthy transition from the law enforcement life.

## Difficult Experiences

After about two months on the job, Brenda experienced one of the most traumatic and horrific incidents of her career.

She was young, enthusiastic, and eager to right the wrongs. She planned to change the world and bring justice to the unjust!

While on patrol, she was flagged down by a couple of kids who told her they had heard shots fired on the other side of the parking lot they were in. She was a rookie, so she was excited. She flew to the other side of the parking lot to see what was going on.

Brenda says she remembers the next part like it happened yesterday. She picked up her radio and said, "Number seven. Be advised I was flagged down by two white males who reported shots fired at..." and she gave the location. The dispatcher came back with, "Number seven, be advised we have a report of an officer in trouble at your location," but the dispatcher didn't click off the radio like they normally did, she held the line open. Then she said, "Number seven, be advised we have a report of an officer down at your location." And that's the last thing Brenda heard before she got out of the car.

As she approached the scene, she saw people huddled around a body on the ground. One man in the huddle turned, and when he did, Brenda could see the victim's pants. They were the same pants she was wearing, and she realized it was someone from the sheriff's office. It was one of her own. He had been killed execution-style. A gunshot wound to the head. Brenda was the first deputy on the scene. She was twenty-four years old.

Soon after this incident, Brenda knew she had been through a traumatic event and wanted to make sure she was okay, so she asked for help. Of course, this was back in a time when there weren't resources available for deputies who were dealing with the mental and emotional fallout from the job. So she was sent to the department guy who was in charge of psychiatric evaluations for pre-hires. He conducted a quick interview and, after checking a few things off on some list, he decided she was okay because she didn't show any of the standard symptoms, like alcoholism, so she was sent on her way.

Therefore, she was on her own to deal with it.

It took Brenda a long time to process what had happened and to reconcile that incident in her head and heart. Many years later, she found herself in that parking lot. She got out of her car and sat on the very same window ledge she had sat on that night, so many years ago, trying to compose herself after that horrific incident. As she sat there reflecting, somewhere deep inside, she knew she was going to be okay.

Later in her career, Brenda was shot at with a twelve-gauge shotgun. The shots missed her, hit the window of her car, and sprayed off. After the shooter was apprehended, he kept screaming at her, "I tried to kill you! I tried to kill you, you fucking sheriff."

I'd like to interject here that my mouth was probably hanging open at this point, because I can't imagine what it's like to have a job so dangerous that you could potentially die on any given day, and I can't fathom what it would be like to face down someone who is *literally* trying to kill you.

I've learned that the examples given here, the stories shared, are the rule and not the exception. First responders see, hear, and endure a lot during their careers. My sincerest gratitude to Brenda for sharing her story with us.

## Turning Point

As Brenda began to think about her inevitable retirement, she decided to try some therapy and just make sure everything was okay. At a certain point in her ongoing therapy, she had an epiphany. She realized that, although she had been meeting with this therapist for quite some time, and she liked her, she hadn't yet allowed herself to fully trust her. She had shared bits and pieces of her story, but not the whole thing.

So, over the course of the next month, Brenda sat down and wrote out twelve pages, in an outline form, of the bigger traumas she had experienced in her life and career. She went all the way back to childhood, and listed those traumas chronologically. At her next counseling appointment, she handed the twelve pages to her therapist and said, "This is my story."

After looking over the pages, the therapist said, "I need to see you once a week for now." Brenda, who up to this point had only popped in every month or two, agreed to switch to weekly sessions. It took four full sessions to go through the twelve pages.

By the end of session two, they had made their way halfway through the list, and Brenda began to dread the third session. Having worked through the first half of her story with the therapist, she remembers thinking, "Maybe I'm too broken to be fixed."

At the onset of the third session, Brenda opened by asking her therapist if she had a plan for what to do with all of this. She began to feel the urgent need to make sure that the therapist had a plan to fix this, to fix her. And the question still lingered: "Am I too broken to be fixed?"

When Brenda looked over the twelve pages she had written, she couldn't imagine that somebody could go through all that and not be broken.

It turns out, she wasn't too broken to be fixed. She wasn't broken at all. But she did need to tell her story, and working through her story with a therapist helped her process all the trauma so she could move forward and eventually retire, healthfully.

# Tools

### Therapy

Brenda admits she was terrified to begin therapy. She had avoided it for a long time, and even carried her therapist's card around for six months before calling to make that first appointment. But she also says it was the best decision she ever made.

For a long time, she kept her therapy appointments a secret, because there was, and still is, a stigma attached to law enforcement officers seeking mental health support. Eventually, people began to find out, and to her surprise, there was acceptance of her choice to go to therapy. Not only that, but her honesty and willingness to be vulnerable and transparent opened the door for others to admit they were in counseling too.

She understands why a lot of people, especially in law enforcement, are resistant to trying therapy. The key, she says, is to find the right therapist, and she knows this is what many first responders dread as they begin to ponder the idea of counseling—the chore of shopping around, and the dread around telling their story to someone who cannot possibly understand what they've been through. Maybe they feel they don't have the time, or they don't want to take the time, to find the right person. Understandably, this process seems tedious and difficult, especially to someone who is dealing with high stress, anxiety, or depression. But this, according to Brenda, is the most important piece. You have to find someone who is a good fit.

### Meditation and Mindfulness

Brenda also cites meditation and mindfulness as crucial tools that help her stay well and balanced. In her words: "Meditation allows me to become a better best friend to myself, more than anything else. It is time spent intensely alone with who I am and who I am in this Universe. Mindfulness has taught me to *feel*, even the benign things...the wind, the cold, etc."

## What Needs to Change

Brenda would love to see embedded therapists in each and every law enforcement organization, or at least, easy access to therapy. She believes that, during annual evaluations, a check-in session with a therapist should be required.

She also believes there needs to be much more mental and emotional preparation provided in the academy, and mandatory, ongoing mental and emotional wellness support and training as the career progresses. This would be an expectation, not an option. She referred to this as Progressive Resilience Training.

> Brenda is a newly retired undersheriff who now runs her own speaking and consulting business, Wayfinder Consulting, LLC.

# • ADAM •

**Fire Service**

Twenty-five years

Started as a volunteer cadet two weeks before his fifteenth birthday; worked up through the ranks

I met Adam in 2017 at a conference where I was teaching meditation and mindfulness to first responders. We chatted during breaks, and I immediately identified him as a super decent human being. His passion for life, his wife and daughter, and his work practically oozes from his pores.

Adam and I live about three hours apart, so we decided to meet on Facetime. I'm intrigued by this man because he is one of those brutally honest people, but in the best possible way. And *he is who he is, unapologetically, all the time.* There is absolutely no bullshit with this guy, and I find that refreshing. We talked for over two and a half hours.

## Difficult Experiences

Adam didn't share a lot of individual stories of traumatic experiences with me. Instead, he talked about the *types* of calls he found most disturbing and upsetting over the years.

He did share one of his earliest memories of a time when he was a cadet, not quite sixteen years old, and worked a massive interior fire. (This would be a big no-no with any department these days.) I simply cannot image a person that age, still a child really, dealing with that level of intensity, trauma, and devastation.

He also spoke eloquently about the emotional toll of being in a leadership role and making decisions on the fly that could potentially get other people injured or killed. There was so much passion and intensity present when Adam spoke about this that I got a little emotional myself.

He told me about a time when he made one such decision and sent people into an extremely dangerous situation. Later, when he reflected on how serious the situation had been, and the weight of the responsibility to make the call he made, he was overcome with emotion. His sense of responsibility for the lives of others is awe-inspiring.

The types of calls that Adam recalled as being especially difficult were infant-not-breathing calls, SIDS deaths, and anything involving children. He said that, when he was younger, he was maybe a little more desensitized and could get into the professional mindset of "just doing his job." But once his own daughter was born, these calls became more challenging and *very* painful.

Another difficult aspect of the job, according to Adam, is the fact that nobody ever talks about the things they see and endure—at least not in a helpful or therapeutic way. "Oh, we talk about it," he said. "But it's usually framed by black humor."

"Black humor" is a term I've heard over and over from first responders. The way these cultures have evolved, it's not okay to talk about the actual incident in a meaningful, emotional way, but it is okay to make a joke.

While this might seem cold or inhuman to some, it is in fact just the opposite, in my opinion. I see it as a human coping mechanism. When a human being witnesses trauma, violence, death, and devastation, but isn't afforded any healthy outlets through which to offload what they've taken in, joking and laughing can serve as a distraction and an emotional release. No human being is built to take on endless trauma and hold onto it.

One more thing that Adam talked to me about was the experience of working on a person, trying to save their life, when you know they aren't going to make it. He shared that this really takes an emotional toll, and is fairly common in his line of work. This one really made me stop and think, or should I say *feel*. I have never experienced, nor can I imagine, trying to save a dying human being, and then watching them die.

When I meet and get to know people like Adam, with this level of depth, passion, and insight, I feel a deep sense of appreciation for the people on this planet who are brave enough and strong enough to live their lives in service to others. I am grateful to Adam for his time, his honesty, and for trusting me.

## Turning Point

When I asked Adam if he had experienced a turning point, there was no hesitation. He said, "I realized that I couldn't continue to drink the amount I was drinking and stay married." He went on to tell me that he also realized he wasn't maintaining as well as he thought he was. He would not have considered himself a person with a drinking *problem*, and he wasn't "technically" an alcoholic, by definition. But he admits that his social drinking was out of control. He was using alcohol as a coping mechanism to numb the emotional pain.

Adam took a class called *Building Resilience and Surviving Secondary Trauma*, taught by Maj. Darren Ivey of the Kansas City, Missouri Police Department. This class was created by a group of people from KCPD and a group from Truman Medical Centers Behavioral Health Center, also located in Kansas City, Missouri. He credits this class as part of the turning point for him. The four-hour block of training takes a deep dive into first-responder stress, trauma, and suicide, and helped Adam put words to what he was experiencing. The data and information contained in the class helped explain why he felt the way he did.

He also learned about the ACE (Adverse Childhood Experiences) test. He took the test and scored very high, meaning he had endured a lot of adverse childhood experiences, which further explained some of the pain and trauma he was carrying.

Adam claims emphatically that his turning point saved his marriage. He says it made him a better father and a better man in every way. Prior to this, he admits that he devalued everything else in his life for the job. That's what he believed. He thought that, in order to be a good firefighter, the job always came first. Now, he prioritizes well-being and family, and he encourages others to do the same.

## Tools

### The Principles of Buddhism and Mindfulness

Along the way, Adam discovered the principles and philosophies of Buddhism and mindfulness. He learned that getting well was an *internal* responsibility and that nothing *external* was going to help him. This discovery led to introspection, and that changed everything.

## What Needs to Change

Adam had a lot to say on this topic, and he made some great points.

"There needs to be less lip service and more action," he said right off the bat. "There needs to be more scientific research on this specific population, this specific culture, and the research needs to be adapted to full-time firefighters versus part-time, and large metropolitan areas versus rural areas."

I asked him what prevents the action. "The stigma. The stigma around mental illness and mental issues and the stigma around having anything wrong with us that we cannot handle."

Adam also noted, "The outside world has changed also. We used to be able to use black humor around the kitchen table; now we are fearful of who will hear and be offended, so we do not share."

In addition to the reduction in sharing, he mentioned the diminished bonding time in recent years. "Many fire departments have individual bedrooms, so when the day is done, firefighters retreat to their private space. We have lost that traditional 'family' time. These changes have impacted our ability to share what bothered us in a way that was culturally accepted in the fire service."

Adam went on to say they need to develop coping programs for recruits, seasoned firefighters, and retirees. The training needs to normalize the aspects of the job that nobody is talking about. I interpreted this as meaning that it needs to address the mental and emotional weight of this profession, not just the critical incidents, in an honest and open way, which will serve to better prepare the recruits, sustain the veterans, and support those who have retired.

He added that the training should educate and inform, must be relevant, and should be regularly updated.

> Adam currently serves his department as Assistant Chief of Training.

# • NATE •

**Military, Law Enforcement**

US Marine Corps, 11th Marines
Counter Battery Radar Platoon

Four years, two combat tours, both in Iraq

Law enforcement, fourteen years

Nate and I sat down in one of my favorite coffee shops in downtown Kansas City so I could interview him for this book. We're both involved with a local organization called The Battle Within, which provides a five-day healing retreat in nature for military veterans and first responders.

Several months ago, Nate and his wife attended one of my four-hour trainings. A few weeks later, he and I met in a barbecue joint to discuss my role with The Battle Within, and I always have the pleasure of seeing him when I teach mindfulness at the retreats. But I first learned of Nate in 2017, when I saw a video clip of him talking about the retreat *he* had attended, that he says saved his life.

Nate is a solid person with an impressive career of service to country and community. He's a big, strong-looking dude with a lot of tattoos, but I get the feeling he's a gentle giant. I've seen his goofy-dad side on social media and it's pretty adorable.

There is something about this guy that is so likeable, and I'm glad to know him. I am grateful to Nate for taking time out of his crazy-busy life to have coffee with me and let me, let us, into his world.

I want to point out that Nate was only seventeen years old when he joined the Marines, and he left for boot camp ten days after turning eighteen. He was deployed to the Middle East twice and was among the first American soldiers to be deployed at the very beginning of the war in 2003.

And here's an eye-popper for you: during his first deployment, he went seventy-six days in the desert without a shower.

## Difficult Experiences

Nate's Counter Battery Radar team was an artillery unit, responsible for tracking enemy shells, mortars, etc. Although they were on the front lines, they never had to fight up close until they hit Baghdad. They set up a headquarters, which the Marines call a CMOC (Civilian-Military Operations Center), and they stood guard around the Sheraton Hotel, located in Baghdad, in the circle where they famously pulled down the statue of Saddam Hussein with a tank.

One night, while Nate was on guard duty, he noticed some movement in the street, and it seemed suspicious. He reported this, and his sergeant instructed him to "put some rounds on it." Shots started to come back at the Marines, which kicked off a massive engagement.

During the gunfight, Nate noticed two individuals approaching, flanking their position, and he fired at them, killing them both.

This incident, Nate says, impacted him more than anything else he ever experienced or endured—the up-close taking of two human lives. He remembers being extremely overwrought and says he *could not* calm himself down. He was in shock. He was shaken to his core. But, instead of offering him some kind of comfort or debrief, his commander pulled him in front of a TV camera.

The journalists were from Turkish CNN, and within minutes of that harrowing incident, they were interviewing Nate on camera. He has no memory of the interview. He was in shock, which had to be clear and apparent to anyone around him. But the shock was never addressed in any way, shape, or form. The kill was glorified. That incident created a deep moral conflict in Nate, which he still lives with to this day.

## Turning Point

The turning point for Nate was a retreat for veterans called Warrior's Ascent. There are so many layers to this story that I wish you could hear him tell it yourself. First of all, he did not want to go, and he was pissed-off to be there. He said a friend of his "rode [him] like a pony," until he finally agreed to go, mostly to shut the guy up.

Nate says he always knew he had post-traumatic stress, but he didn't know it was affecting his life. He thought it was just something he had to deal with. He says, "I was angry. I was always angry. I was cold." He says he considered being "hard" to be a good thing. He didn't feel things. He didn't cry when he was sad. Admittedly, he was locked-up inside.

So there was nothing about this retreat that appealed to him. He thought it was "hippie bullshit," and he simply did not think he needed it.

But surprisingly, once there, he changed his opinion pretty quickly and began to think there might be something in it for him after all.

One of his most profound moments came toward the end of the retreat. There is a ceremony in the woods that all the attendees participate in, and he was helping clean up afterward. He grabbed a water cooler and started carrying it to one of the cars. As he emerged from the woods, he says he looked around, and he could see colors that he felt like he'd never seen before. The wind felt different on his skin. The clouds looked crisper in the sky. He stopped and wondered, "What the hell is this?" He didn't know what was happening.

He brought this up with one of the counselors later, who told him, "You've literally suppressed your emotions and feelings for so long that your body has suppressed your physical senses."

Nate calls that realization his "big 'holy crap' moment." He realized this was truly a new beginning for him. He says, without that retreat, he would not be married, and it helped him become a much better dad.

## Tools

### Meditation

Nate cited meditation as the number-one tool that helped him heal and continues to help him on his healing path. He has meditated nearly every day for five years now. He told me, "It helps me slow the 'busy' me down so I can *observe* the problem instead of *being in the problem*."

As a side note, Nate added that he was born with a stutter, and meditation has helped his stutter tremendously. He notices that, when he skips meditation, the stutter gets worse.

### Therapy

Therapy is another important tool that helped Nate. He initially tried therapy in several different ways, and he also tried medications. That path, he said, was even more traumatizing, because he couldn't find the right therapist and it felt like nothing was working. After the retreat, he was finally able to find a therapist with whom he could connect. That's when therapy began to help.

## Community

Nate says community is an important element of healing for him, and his community helps him maintain his growth. And, he says, developing the ability to be vulnerable has also been a key component to his well-being.

## What Needs to Change

When I asked Nate this question, right off the bat, he said, "The whole 'John Wayne' thing needs to die. It made good movies, but it's not real."

He went on to say that nobody should ever be shamed for admitting that something's wrong and they're trying to work through it. He added that, in the military and in law enforcement, it is frowned upon to ask for help, and that has to stop. Also, in his experience, there needs to be better integration of the business side and the personal side of military and law enforcement operations.

> Nate currently serves as a police officer with a metropolitan police department and is the Program Director for The Battle Within, Kansas City.

# • DAWN •

## Dispatch

Twenty-five years

Served as a clerk, a call taker, a dispatcher,
and a dispatch supervisor

I first met Dawn in 2017 when she attended one of my classes at a local mental health center. She introduced herself, and we chatted about how much meditation and mindfulness could help call takers and dispatchers. Then, in January of 2019, Dawn attended my train-the-trainer class to learn more about teaching Learn to Pause Mindfulness Training and Pause15 Meditation.

Dawn is a fierce advocate for dispatchers and a big believer that meditation and mindfulness instruction should be offered to all telecommunicators.

I have so much respect for this strong, compassionate woman, and I just really like her. She has endured a tremendous amount of trauma in her life, both personally and professionally. I'd like to allow Dawn to tell you about that in her own words.

## Difficult Experiences

"As a supervisor, it is my job to listen to and make copies of 911 calls and dispatch air traffic for any critical incident. I have heard shots being fired at officers. I've listened as an officer's radio mike was stuck because he was being dragged down the highway by a vehicle driven by a drunk driver. I've listened as an officer was screaming because he couldn't find his partner who had been hit by a car while throwing out stop sticks.

"I have listened to people being raped and parents who have woken up after rolling over on their infant who is no longer breathing. I've experienced [schizophrenic] people changing personalities over the phone. I have listened to people begging us to find them, even though they had no idea where they were, and some of those people ended up dying because we couldn't find them. I have listened to people scream for help because their loved one was shot, and I've listened as that loved one took their last breath."

As I reread Dawn's words, I am shocked and saddened by what these brave professionals endure.

I'd like to interject here and share that I visited Dawn a few months ago at the dispatch center where she has worked for twenty-five years. She gave me a tour of the call-taker side and the dispatch side of operations. Then she and I took a seat next to one of the dispatchers so I could observe. Within minutes, a call came in that I will never forget. When I got home, I wrote the following recap on my PauseFirst Project Facebook page:

March 30, 2019

I recently visited a large metropolitan dispatch center. I was blown away by all the activity and the skill and professionalism of the dispatchers. They graciously showed me around and described the process of taking calls and dispatching officers. And then a call came in that I will never forget.

Motionless, I observed as this call unfolded. At first, I could only hear the dispatcher's side of the conversation: suicide attempt.

Fourteen-year-old boy. Gunshot wound to the head. Caller attempting CPR.

Then a supervisor made the call audible, and I could hear the caller. The boy's mother.

The desperate screams of a mother trying to save her child hit my ears like a lightning bolt, and I began to cry. I had to leave the room. I was shaken to my core, and I cry as I relive and recount this event.

I could write an entire book about the experience, but here's the crux of what I wish to convey:

1. *Dispatchers are first responders.*

2. I am deeply grateful to all emergency responders. They see, hear, and endure untold tragedy on a daily basis.

3. I will continue to work hard to raise awareness about first-responder stress, trauma, secondary trauma, and suicide.

4. **As a society, we need to do a much better job of caring for our first responders. They are traumatized.**

What in the world would we do without these brave people? Who would protect, save, and rescue us? They run toward danger and devastation while the rest of us are running away.

There's one more thing I'd like you to consider about the dispatcher who took this call. Unlike me, she couldn't cry. She couldn't walk out. She *can't* walk away. Why? Because, as the officers and emergency medical techs arrive on the scene, there's another call coming in, and she has to take it.

Side note: Sadly, in most states, dispatchers are not classified as first responders; they are classified as "clerical." In Dawn's words, "Call takers and dispatchers are the *first* first responders."

Now, bearing in mind Dawn's professional stress and trauma, let's continue by hearing from her what she has experienced personally.

> "In 2016, after a four-year battle with drug addiction and mental illness, my twenty-three-year-old daughter committed suicide. I happened to be the one to find her. She also used my weapon to complete the suicide. I had to be the one to tell my fifteen-year-old twin sons their sister had died. This absolutely turned my world upside down.

> "Since then, in February of 2019, I also lost my brother-in-law to suicide. He was an undercover police officer at the time. I was with my sister when she found out. She is now a single mother of three boys, one of whom is the son of the police officer.

> "Currently, one of my sons is working through his own depression and anxiety as a result of these traumas in our personal life."

I want to thank Dawn for her raw vulnerability, and for letting us into her world. Her story helps highlight the fact that first responders, who deal with indescribable stress and trauma at work every day, also experience stress and trauma in their personal lives, just like the rest of us. As a society, we need to raise awareness of this fact, and proactively find ways to help and support these fine people.

# Turning Point

Dawn shared that her turning point occurred in 2017. While she was working, a call came in reporting that a female had jumped off a bridge into the Missouri River. Officers were dispatched and were able to rescue the woman and take her to the hospital for treatment.

A few hours later, dispatch received a call from a man who said he had just returned home from work and found that his eight-year-old son had been drowned in the bathtub.

It turned out these two calls were related. The woman who had jumped from the bridge earlier was the mother of this boy, and she was the one who had drowned him.

Remember, in the previous year, Dawn had lost her daughter to suicide. What you don't know is that Dawn found her daughter in the bathtub, having completed suicide. So the incident with the mother and the boy and the bathtub, understandably, triggered a tremendous amount of trauma for Dawn.

After this incident, Dawn decided to attend the West Coast Post-Trauma Retreat (WCPR), a program designed for first responders whose lives have been affected by their work experience.

# Tools

Dawn found the West Coast Post-Trauma Retreat to be very helpful. She says it was comforting to know that she wasn't being judged for what she was going through, and she felt supported by everyone there.

## EMDR

One of the most impactful experiences during the WCPR, according to Dawn, was EMDR therapy. EMDR stands for eye movement desensitization and reprocessing.

Dawn says, "Prior to EMDR, the memory of finding my daughter was very vivid. The colors were vivid, the scene was very large and seemed very close to me. After EMDR, there was a complete change. The mental image—the picture—seemed far away and small. It was softened, like it had a cloud over it."

EMDR is proving to be an effective treatment for first responders who are dealing with post-traumatic stress symptoms and/or a diagnosis of PTSD (post-traumatic stress disorder).

## Meditation and Breathing Techniques

Dawn also cites meditation and breathing as important tools she uses every day. She says, "When I feel myself getting stressed or worked up, I stop what I'm doing and take a short break to breathe. Deep breaths do wonders to get me back on track."

## Coloring

Believe it or not, Dawn has found coloring to be extremely relaxing, and it is a tool she says she uses almost every night before going to bed.

## Therapy

Dawn also included therapy in the list of tools she has found helpful on her healing path. She says she sees a therapist regularly.

## What Needs to Change

According to Dawn, first and foremost, we must let first responders know it's okay to not be okay. She says the "suck it up buttercup" days need to end because human beings are not built to see, hear, and endure the things that first responders encounter on a daily basis.

Here are a few more of Dawn's suggestions:

- Have resources available to first responders when they need someone to talk to, and *this must be someone they can trust.*

- Create peer support teams.

- Have therapists available to work with first responders in crisis, and ensure that these therapists specialize in treating first responders.

---

Dawn currently serves as a Dispatch Supervisor for a metropolitan police department.

She co-facilitates CIT (Crisis Intervention Training) for telecommunicators.

She has participated in the WCPR Retreat in a peer support role.

She is part of a roving peer support team for call takers and dispatchers.

And she is on the advisory committee and is a team leader for her department's Peer Support Team.

---

# • JOHN •

**Law Enforcement**

Twenty years

Police Officer, Police Sergeant

John and I met in 2017 after a mindfulness presentation I delivered at a local police academy. He introduced himself and told me the short version of his story, and we talked for a long time as we packed up and walked to our cars. He's so darn easy to talk to.

John has an authenticity and sweetness about him that is magnetic. When you meet him, you want to be his friend. We've stayed in touch, and we've seen each other here and there in the past two years. I knew, as I started to formulate ideas for this book, that I wanted to interview John.

## Difficult Experiences

When John was seventeen years old, his big brother committed suicide. The brothers were only fifteen months apart in age. "We were best friends," John told me. "That was a devastating loss."

I can attest to the fact that there is no loss like suicide. It leaves a massive hole. I'm not saying it's worse than other losses, just different. Suicide is unique because it is incredibly difficult to live with the fact that a person you loved was in so much pain that they did not want to live. In a way, suicide passes that pain onto survivors.

Next, John told me about another devastating blow. Two and a half years into policing, a good friend of his, a fellow officer who had been on the job a very long time, died in a line-of-duty shooting. John says this officer was a veteran when John was new to the job, and he was the only "old-timer" who would talk to him in his rookie days. In some ways, John recalls, the older officer felt "fatherly." His death hit hard.

Aside from the day-to-day stress and trauma that police officers encounter on the job, such as violent individuals, intoxicated people who want to fight, drug overdoses, brutal domestic violence, and crimes against children, most of them are also suffering with invisible wounds and pain, like John was. John now realizes he was carrying unprocessed trauma that reached back into his childhood and continued to pile up throughout his adulthood and career.

## Turning Point

What John shared with me about his turning point is both heartbreaking and inspirational. As you know, my husband's suicide was the catalyst for the work I'm doing now, and I'm sure you're also aware that law enforcement suicide is epidemic and getting worse. This story, from a veteran cop who wanted to die, came very close to dying, but ultimately survived and is thriving, encapsulates the entire purpose of this book.

I am so grateful to John for his vulnerability.

John shared that, just a few years ago, he was sitting in his truck in a parking lot, "ugly-crying," and trying to muster the courage to put his gun in his mouth and pull the trigger. He had made the decision to take his own life, he had a plan, and he was prepared to execute that plan. His phone, on the seat next to him, had been ringing and ringing, but he was ignoring it. Then, all of a sudden, he got a text, and for some reason he decided to look at it. It was a supportive text from a friend, and something about that text sort of "snapped him out of it," as he recalls.

Two weeks later, knowing he was in desperate need of support, John attended a five-day retreat in nature, which was designed for military veterans and first responders. That retreat changed John's life forever.

I want to take a moment and reflect on how close John came to dying by his own hand. He was so traumatized, unhappy, and hopeless that he believed death was the only way to escape the pain. If this resonates with you even a little, please know this: John's life looks nothing like it did just a couple of years ago. He is happy, he is fulfilled, he has love in his life, he takes good care of himself, he is a better dad, and he is leading, mentoring, and teaching others.

If you feel none of this is possible for you, please understand that John once felt none of it was possible for him either. But he didn't pull that trigger. He reached out for help and he rebuilt himself from the inside out. Today, John is truly happy. Believe me, I've known him for two years now, and we spent a very long time catching up in that coffee shop. The dude is living his best life.

## Tools

### Meditation

John says his number-one wellness tool, hands-down, is meditation. He learned how to meditate at the retreat he attended, and he began to use meditation to help him identify and control his responses to the emotions he was feeling.

John continues to meditate. In fact, he recently hit an important goal. John meditated every single day, without exception, for three hundred sixty-fix days! One year of meditation, no missed days. That's pretty impressive!

He says meditation has made him much more mindful in his life.

### Therapy

John says therapy has been a life-saver for him, but he cautions others, "You've got to find the right therapist and you have to open up, or it won't help."

# What Needs to Change

John says we have to make it okay for police officers and other first responders to show their emotions in a healthy way. He says the law enforcement culture has done a lot of harm by teaching people to be non-emotional. In his opinion, there is strength in showing emotion in the proper way at the proper time.

Also, he's adamant that asking for help must become acceptable, because, he says, people are masking and numbing their pain with alcohol, prescription drugs, and sex.

According to John, cops are trained to suggest that people seek professional help for mental and emotional struggles, but they don't take their own advice. He thinks recruits need to understand how bad things will be, and they must be encouraged to make themselves a priority. "You can't devote your life to helping everyone but yourself," John says.

He also believes that recruits in the academy need to be told the truth about the job in a more direct way. He says they need to hear things like, "You're going to see the worst of humanity. Friends are going to die. You will be in danger, regularly." Then, John says, "Veteran cops should come in and tell their stories to emphasize these realities."

John also feels mental and emotional training should be integrated into the academy to better prepare recruits for what they will witness and endure.

> John is currently a Police Sergeant with a
> metropolitan police department.

# • WENDY •

**Law Enforcement**

Twenty-two years

Special Agent, INS (now DHS—
Department of Homeland Security)

Police Officer, Detective

Substance Abuse Coordinator, Sheriff's Department

Wendy and I met in 2017 at a CIT (Crisis Intervention Team) meeting where I was teaching mindfulness. We had an instant connection, primarily because she is so dang easy to like. After that meeting, we stayed in touch and have become friends, even though we live three hours apart. The more I learn about Wendy's life path and career, the more impressed I am.

## Difficult Experiences

In Wendy's career, she has primarily worked Crimes Against Persons, including homicide, gangs, domestic violence, and sex crimes.

Wendy started this conversation by sharing that, in her early days as a police officer, working third shift, she encountered a lot of difficulty with male coworkers. (I'm so glad she brought this up because it's prevalent among female law enforcement, and like everything else we're addressing in this book, needs to be brought to light.) The men, she says, treated her very poorly, and that added a tremendous amount of unnecessary stress to an already stressful job.

Another crucially important aspect Wendy cited was balancing motherhood and her career. Both of her daughters were born prematurely, which adds mightily to the stressors of parenthood. She remembers one day in particular, getting a call at work that her infant daughter was sick and needed to be picked up immediately. Wendy's husband, also law enforcement, was not available, and although Wendy was extremely busy at work, she had to leave.

Driving home that day with her infant daughter in tow, the intense stress of the situation got the best of Wendy, and she had a panic attack, something she had never experienced before. The panic attack was so intense, she says, that she could barely breathe and had to pull the car over.

Something else Wendy addressed, which nobody else in this book mentioned, is organizational stress. In my many interactions and private conversations with first responders over the years, I can attest to the fact that this is a primary stressor. People often share with me that bosses, supervisors, outdated policies, power struggles, and bureaucracy contribute hugely to their stress.

On top of all of this, remember, there is the day-to-day stress and trauma of police work.

Early in Wendy's career, she worked with a domestic violence victim who was later killed by the perpetrator who had abused her. After trying to help this victim and getting to know her and her story, the woman's death hit Wendy very hard.

At another point in Wendy's career, she worked a serial rapist case that for her, as a woman, was extremely difficult.

Another tough case that really hit home involved a little girl whose mother had been killed by her boyfriend. The girl was the one who found her mother, shot in the head. This was a gut-wrenching interview because, at the time, Wendy's own daughter was the same age as the little girl. As the girl described what she'd experienced, Wendy says she had to fight hard to hold back her own emotions. She remembers going home, hugging her daughter, and then talking to her husband about what had happened.

I'm going to interject here with an observation. I believe the last few words of that last sentence are critical: *she talked to her husband about what had happened*. I have discovered that this is a missing component for nearly every first responder. They are traumatized, they have endured horrors most of us can't imagine, but they don't talk about any of it.

This culture of silent suffering has got to change. *Talking* about one's stress, trauma, and experiences is an important step to processing and healing from the exposure to them. Nobody is built to take on years of trauma and hold it in.

## Turning Point

Wendy says, looking back, even though she loved her job and was happy at home, she was drowning in guilt. When she was at work, she felt she should be at home. When she was at home, she felt she should be working. She realizes in hindsight that she existed in a constant state of fight or flight, and she didn't sleep well for over a decade.

At the age of forty-one, Wendy tried yoga for the first time, primarily as a way to lose residual baby weight. Unexpectedly, she says, she noticed that she started to feel better overall. She felt calmer and more patient, even when she wasn't doing yoga. She admits yoga was not an instant fix, but it was the first step on her path to healing.

## Tools

### Yoga

Wendy's number-one wellness tool is yoga. "It's my go-to physical activity that allows me to incorporate breathing and mindfulness," she says. Wendy is a two-hundred-hour RYT (Registered Yoga Teacher) and a YFFR (Yoga for First Responders) Ambassador.

### Breathwork

"Breathwork is my go-to because it's accessible anywhere, anytime."

### Meditation

"Since I started to meditate regularly about two years ago, I have fine-tuned my self-awareness. Allowing myself to sit with discomfort and learning to recognize my triggers have been very helpful in all aspects of my life."

### Therapy

Wendy also listed therapy as one of her wellness tools.

### Talking to Friends

There was a time when Wendy kept everything very close and only talked to her husband about her experiences. Now she calls "talking to friends" her version of peer support. Once she was firmly planted on a healing path, she began opening up and discussing things with trusted friends. She says having a good, solid support system is extremely helpful.

## What Needs to Change

Wendy is a firm believer that we must begin to normalize the conversation regarding issues that law enforcement officers, and other first responders, face. She feels that every department should have a comprehensive wellness program to include peer support, family support, resilience training (mindfulness, emotional intelligence), and embedded psychologists.

She points out that, in 2017, Congress passed the LEMHWA (Law Enforcement Mental Health and Wellness Act), which offers grant funding for peer support, resilience training, and more. She believes recognition of the importance of these issues at the federal level is necessary, and that it will trickle down to local government.

In Wendy's own experience, introducing yoga to her department and initiating a conversation about wellness and mindfulness has been impactful. She's noticed a significant shift in mindset.

She admits that introducing yoga into the law enforcement culture was not easy, and there was a lot of pushback in the beginning, but that has improved immensely. She says she admires the leadership at the time for allowing the implementation of the yoga program, which they offered internally and also taught to recruits.

In terms of what needs to change, this example points to leadership. The people at the top have to begin embracing new approaches to wellness. Officer mental and emotional well-being must be prioritized, and the culture must evolve into one of balance and holistic care for the men and women who wear the uniform, and all who surround and support them.

Wendy now serves as the Substance Abuse Coordinator for her local Sheriff's Department.

# • MYRONE •

**Law Enforcement**

Sixteen years

Police Officer, Police Sergeant

This guy. Oh my goodness. Myrone, pronounced "Myron." A one-of-a-kind spelling for a one-of-a-kind man.

I've gotten to know Myrone over the past couple of years, and I consider him a friend. He's realer than real. He is who he is, unapologetically. He's a thinker. He studies life and lives fully. He's just a solid human being.

Myrone came to one of my classes back in 2017. He spoke up in class and talked to the group about his struggles with anxiety and how he came to find meditation. He was funny—he's a storyteller—but he was also genuine, and he piqued my curiosity. I was impressed with the way he opened up and shared so easily. This, I can assure you, is not the norm in my first-responder classes.

Several months later, Myrone allowed me to visit him at work and interview him on video about his experiences with job stress and anxiety and his thoughts about meditation for first responders. Then, in January of this year, he attended my train-the-trainer class. We've stayed in touch and we're connected on social media, and that's where I really see him shine. Myrone likes to stir the pot and make people think and feel. He's not really a shit-starter, he's more of a conversation starter.

One thing I greatly admire about Myrone is his dedication to family. He is laser-focused on being the best version of himself, and he's committed to being a good man, husband, and father. He realizes this takes effort, so he works on himself to help keep the family unit strong. This, to me, is epic!

## Difficult Experiences

Myrone shared an experience that occurred early in his career, which made him realize for the first time, in a very real way, that his job is dangerous. He was on duty in a patrol car, like so many nights before, when a call went out about a house fire.

He and another officer drove toward the address to see how they might be able to assist. As he approached the street, he could see a massive neighborhood fire blazing, something he had never seen before. He parked his car and ran toward the scene. The fire, he recalls, had engulfed the entire house, and as he approached, he could feel the intense heat radiating.

Bystanders on-scene indicated that people were trapped in the back of the house, so Myrone ran to the back. He broke down the back door and found an elderly man, just inside the doorway. The man was holding an infant and had been trying to get out, but the heat, flames and black smoke had prevented him from exiting.

Myrone grabbed the baby girl from the man's arms and handed her off to someone, then began performing CPR on the older gentleman. As he tried to save the man, he realized he was dangerously close to the fire and needed to move away. He picked the man up and ran with him to a safer distance and continued to try to revive him. He was finally able to carry the man to an ambulance parked down the street. Unfortunately, the man did not survive.

In fact, five people died that night—the elderly man, his infant granddaughter, and three other grandchildren.

Myrone was taken to the hospital and treated for smoke inhalation. He says he was very shaken-up as the reality of the dangerous nature of his job began to sink in. At the time, two of his children were the same ages as two of the children who died. That was something that hit him hard.

In my experience with first responders, this is a common experience—working calls that involve children the same age as, or with similarities to, their own children. Many have shared with me how emotionally wrenching this is, and how it creates fear and hypervigilance in them. They can't stop thinking, "That could have been *my* child."

As Myrone recounts this story, he says, "I can still remember it like it was yesterday. I can feel the heat, smell the smoke..."

He says he never spoke with a chaplain, there was no EAP (employee assistance program), and he did not seek help to process the experience. He just powered on. Because that's what he believed he was supposed to do.

## Turning Point

Around the time Myrone got promoted to sergeant, he also found out he and his wife were expecting their third child, and his mother passed away. He says he also encountered "a whole bunch of other life and job stuff," all at the same time, and for *the first time in his life*, Myrone began to experience the uncomfortable and sometimes debilitating symptoms of anxiety.

He shared with me that the anxiety got so bad, he was struggling to function normally, and he literally felt like he was dying. "But," he said, "nobody knew. I was really good at hiding it, and I could always work."

When I asked him how bad things got, he said, "I never actually thought about suicide, but I did occasionally think the world might be better off without me, and I would wonder what it would it be like if I just died."

It was a marriage issue that motivated Myrone to try therapy during this time, and that decision turned out to be his turning point. Talking to the therapist led him to open up about job stress and, for the first time, with the help of the therapist, he realized he had PTSD.

He gained awareness, through therapy, that job-related stress combined with adverse childhood experiences caused the PTSD, and he faced the fact that it was all catching up with him. The therapist helped him work through these issues and offered tools, including meditation, to help him navigate the anxiety. This was his real breakthrough, he says—learning how to meditate and committing to a meditation practice.

## Tools

Myrone quickly ticked off a short, definite list when I asked him about the tools he uses to stay healthy and balanced.

"Self-care, working out, eating a decently healthy diet, and meditation."

## What Needs to Change

He was also very definite with his answers to this question.

It took him no time at all to shoot back, "Cops need to stop hiding behind their badge. They need to be real." He went on to say, "We think we have all the answers. We have the solutions for everyone else, but we won't apply those solutions to ourselves."

I asked him what he would say to an officer on the fence, someone who is struggling but hasn't reached out for help. His answer was direct. "You are responsible for your own well-being."

Myrone believes the onus is on the individual, and they must take the scary steps and do the hard work to get well and healthy, for themselves and for their families and the people they love.

Myrone, thank you for your open honesty, and for being a positive role model for others. You're a good dude.

> Myrone currently serves as a Police Sergeant for a metropolitan police department.

# • ANGELA •

**Military, Fire Service**

United States Air Force, reservist
for almost twenty years

Six overseas deployments to the Middle East

EMT, Paramedic, Fire Service EMS,
twenty-two years

EMS Lieutenant

Aeromedical Evacuation Technician

Certified Flight Communicator and
Transport Medical Technician

I had the pleasure of meeting Angela shortly after she was promoted to training officer with a local metropolitan fire department. One of her chiefs knew that she and I shared an interest in meditation and mindfulness, so he facilitated the connection. We met in a coffee shop and I liked her right away. Her intelligence is almost intimidating, and she's impressively articulate. But her warmth and sincerity lend a humility that makes her easy to be with and likeable. I love talking to her. I always learn something.

Angela came to my house one evening after work so I could interview her for this book. We dined on veggies and hummus and fruit and cheese while we visited and talked about her impressive career and the jaw-dropping things she has seen and done in her twenty-plus years of service.

# Difficult Experiences

Angela's story begins when she was only eighteen. She grew up in Oklahoma City, and while she was still in high school, she signed up to volunteer for a search and rescue organization. She took CPR and first aid classes in high school, and she says she always felt drawn to that kind of work.

I could not believe my ears when she told me what her first big volunteer experience was. It was the Oklahoma City bombing. Now, remember, she was still in high school.

Angela said she went to the location of the bombing with a dust mask, gloves, and a flashlight. When she arrived on the scene, she saw lines of people—rescuers of all kinds—waiting to get in the building and help. She got in line, entered the building, and began searching—digging around in the rubble, feeling for bodies. Whenever she came upon a body, she immediately went about trying to determine if it was dead or alive. In two full days of searching, Angela did not find one person who had survived. She found bodies, just no survivors.

When I asked her about the shock and trauma of the situation, she admitted it was pretty terrible. She says she was offered some form of debriefing on-scene by a psychology student, but she declined.

After graduating, Angela went to college for a couple of years, but admittedly didn't do very well. During those years, she noticed a lot of residual issues stemming from the bombing. She was having nightmares and persistent thoughts about the event. It became a preoccupation. She followed all the news about Timothy McVeigh and Terry Nichols, the then-suspects, and she drove by the site often.

While in college, Angela says she sought counseling, but she didn't feel it helped. She says there was no resonance with the therapist, so she gave up. Looking back, she realizes she felt numb for a very long time.

Angela went on to join the Air Force as a reservist. During her service, she was deployed to the Middle East *six* times. She worked as a flight medic on a C-130 aircraft and was an Aeromedical Evacuation Technician Flight Instructor/Examiner.

I asked her what that experience was like—being on an aircraft in a war zone, landing in dangerous places, evacuating and transporting wounded soldiers. She told me the planes got shot at a lot, by rifles, missiles, and mortars. This, of course, was stressful and traumatic, but just part of the job. She also told me about a harrowing experience on base one night.

In one single night, from sunup to sundown, thirty-six mortars hit the base where Angela was stationed. She said it was nonstop, so much so that she began trying to calculate her odds of surviving the night. I can't imagine how scary that must have been, how terrifying and traumatic. I realize that this is the reality of war—this is what war is, what war does—but that realization doesn't make it okay. At least, not to me. We need to do a much better job of caring for people when they return home from these awful experiences.

In my opinion, we as a society have simply not paid enough attention to what our men and women in uniform endure. There has not been nearly enough understanding of the trauma, and therefore not enough empathy, support, and healing for these

The Mindfulness for Warriors Handbook

people who put their lives on the line and, in the process, see, hear, and experience unimaginable devastation, destruction, and death. No human being is built to withstand this.

Angela has since lost multiple friends, many to suicide. One friend drank herself to death. Another died of brain cancer, likely due to injury and physical damage incurred in her job as a military firefighter. And yet another died in a helicopter crash later, after he had returned to civilian life.

That's yet another tragic commonality among military veterans. On top of the death and devastation they see, they also lose a lot of friends in the course of war—and afterward—to suicide, fatal injuries, illnesses, and ailments.

Now, add to Angela's traumatic military experiences her twenty-two years of working as an EMT and paramedic. Emergency medical personnel see and deal with heinous injuries, devastating loss, life-and-death situations, and tragedies most of us can't even imagine.

With all this in mind, I asked Angela a pointed question: Knowing what you know now, would you take a different path?

Her answer came quickly, and it was emphatic. "No," she said. "I would still sign up."

Are you familiar with that popping-eye emoji? I'm pretty sure that's what I looked like when she said those words.

But here's what she shared with me. She said she always felt like this work was a fit for her. She said when she was younger, she couldn't quite explain why, but then she learned something from a psychologist she met after deployment.

He said, if anyone ever implies that you are an adrenaline junkie—addicted to the rush of adrenaline this job gives you, I want you to remember this. You are not addicted to adrenaline; you are addicted to *relevance*. RELEVANCE.

Whew! Let that one sink in for a minute.

Here's the thing. I think this is prevalent among first responders. I believe many of them get into these professions to help others, as cliché as that might be. In my experience, a great number of these people feel a pull or a calling or whatever you want to call it. They *need* to help, to be of service, and to lend their natural skills and abilities to the greater good. There is something inside them that drives them to duty and service—to *relevance*—to knowing they are somehow making a difference in this world.

As I type, my body is covered in goosebumps and my eyes are teary, because I feel such respect and appreciation for these people. They sacrifice a part of themselves for us, and I am deeply grateful.

## Turning Point

Angela cites lots of little turning points along the way, but can pinpoint some key components that led to healing. I'll let Angela tell you in her own words.

> "Certainly, there were many things that led to where I am today. I am seeing more and more of my life as connected and recognizing that every part of my history, including all the challenges and triumphs, is the foundation of each subsequent moment. One particularly catalyzing moment was when I heard Joan Halifax teaching about having what is called a 'strong back and soft front.' This

is the characterization of someone who is vulnerable, allowing their heart to be accessible in deeply caring for others as well as revealing their authentic self, while simultaneously embodying strength and capability. I was fascinated by this idea because I had seen the two—strength and vulnerability—as being opposed. It was the typical cultural understanding, particularly in first-responder culture.

"I took on a sort of experiment in my life and began to reveal to trusted friends, as well as a therapist, what my experiences had been and how I had (or in many cases *had not*) been processing those intense parts of my life and career. What I found in this exploration is that the most important people in my life didn't find these conversations nearly as distressing as I thought they might. They were interested, but not overly so, and they cared about me. They also knew that I cared about them and it was safe to share their own vulnerabilities with me. We connected, not in spite of my thoughts and feelings, but because of them. Shockingly, no one reacted as though I was weak or broken.

"Cultivating a 'strong back' didn't require the intentionality of accessing my 'soft front.' I found that opening up to myself and others didn't wreck me in the way I worried it would. It wasn't the opening of the floodgates for all my suffering which would leave me drowned and helpless. It didn't break me to begin feeling what actually was present in my mind, body, and spirit. Instead, it revealed that, although I am tender-hearted and have some difficult emotions, there is also a breadth of happiness and love that I was unable to experience when I was closed-off.

It's the experience of emotion and the capacity to share it that connects people, and this connection is so needed for healing."

# Tools

## Therapy

Angela says she eventually found a good therapist, and therapy has been hugely helpful. She emphasizes that there *are* good therapists and you *can* find one. But, she says, you have to be ready. She also added, if a person finds themself wanting to explore therapy, they should not be discouraged by having to go through three or four therapists in order to find the right one. This might just be part of the process and will be well worth the effort.

## Meditation

"Meditation has saved my life." These are Angela's words. "It has given me the ability to respond and not just react, react, react. It paved the way for all of the healing."

## Veteran's PATH
## (Peace, Acceptance, Transformation, Honor)

Attending a program based on meditation, mindfulness, and physical and outdoor experiences, provided by the organization known as Veteran's PATH, was a crucial step on Angela's healing path. "Veteran's PATH changed my life," she said.

## Telling My Story

Angela included one more important step on her healing path: "Telling my story. Vulnerability."

*This* is huge, and it's the reason I wrote the book. Angela is wrapping up this segment of the book because she ended where I began—storytelling—the importance of sharing our stories so that others don't feel so alone.

## What Needs to Change

Angela believes first responders must be able to start telling their stories, and to do that, they have to let go of the idea that their story is so unique that nobody will understand, or that nobody wants to hear it, or that telling the story will put the burden on others.

She perfectly conveys the unspoken and underlying rhetoric that keeps first responders from speaking up.

"We don't need to be taken care of by others. We don't *need* help, we *are the help*," Angela shared. "But that needs to change," she went on. "We need to see ourselves as worthy of receiving the support that's being offered."

This is such powerful insight! Another component that keeps first responders silent is fear—fear of stigma, fear of being judged—even fear of being demoted or dismissed. Historically, it has not been acceptable to admit to mental or emotional distress in these cultures.

Because first responders are our heroes—our savers and rescuers—they sometimes feel they must project invincibility. Sharing their stories means letting down their guard, and that requires vulnerability. Vulnerability has traditionally been seen as a weakness in first-responder professions, so people stay quiet, and suffer in silence.

While writing an article about my husband's suicide for *In Public Safety* online, I had my own epiphany about vulnerability as I struggled to honestly share my experiences with David's mental and emotional problems and how they affected our marriage. After sending the article to my editor, I felt a rush of panic, and I recognized this feeling as vulnerability. It was scary and uncomfortable to let my own guard down and speak the truth.

That experience led me to a deeper understanding of what first responders live with. I had nothing to lose in sharing my story, it just made me feel exposed. But first responders believe they have a lot to lose, and whether it's real or perceived, that belief prevents them from accepting the help that's available. This has to change. First responders must be allowed to tell their stories and seek help without fear of ridicule or retribution, which will require both individual courage and cultural evolution.

I am so grateful to Angela for *her* willingness to be vulnerable and share her story with us.

> Angela now serves as a Training Officer for
> her department.

# WHAT I'VE LEARNED

In my work with first responders, and through my interactions with the nine brave souls you just read about, I've noticed some common threads. The observations I'm about to share stem from my time with first responders in the classroom, my participation in first-responder healing retreats, my friendships and relationships with first responders, and my time spent with these interviewees. I am not saying that every first responder has experienced or exhibits every one of these traits, but I've learned that these are some commonalities.

## They All Suffer

This is the only commonality I can say categorically applies to each and every first responder and veteran. As a society, we have underestimated and glossed over the suffering of our active-duty military personnel, dispatchers, police, firefighters, paramedics, EMTs, social workers, military veterans, emergency techs, clergy, ER personnel, nurses, doctors, and others.

These people encounter, see, hear, endure, and are impacted by the trauma of others on a regular and ongoing basis. Yes, they are strong, skilled, and brave individuals. But they are also human beings with the same emotional systems the rest of us have. Don't think for one second that any of these people are "built for this work." The fact that they are capable and heroic doesn't mean they don't feel pain or cry tears.

They are compassionate, and they possess empathy. If you know a first responder who is "hard," or seems cold or distant, know that that is a mask, a protection mechanism, or a survival tactic. Don't let them fool you. They are hurting and they're terrified to let their guard down. See the humanity in them, give them the grace of your compassion and understanding, and do what you can to help.

No human being is built to endure the stress, pain, trauma, and suffering of a first responder. They all suffer.

## Many Experienced Childhood Trauma

It might surprise you to know that a high percentage of people who go into the helping (first-responder) professions do so partly because of childhood trauma. Many have reported experiencing rough, dysfunctional, neglectful, and sometimes abusive childhoods. Not all, but some, of the folks I interviewed shared with me that their childhoods were not ideal, to say the least.

Often people who endured adverse childhood experiences will seek out professions that allow them the opportunity to help others and right the wrongs.

I include this information in order to point out that the first responders who had traumatic childhoods are carrying *that* trauma on top of the trauma of the job. Remember earlier, when I talked about *accumulated* stress and trauma? If childhood pain and dysfunction is not properly processed and healed, it simply piles up.

## Shame Is an Epidemic

There's a recurring theme among first responders, and it is shame. For some, shame originated in childhood or early life when they were victimized or abused. For others, it developed over time, throughout their career, as they struggled to cover up how they felt inside. Some people feel shame because they aren't as resilient as they used to be, and feel themselves succumbing to the symptoms of stress, anxiety, and depression. Still others carry shame based on their actions and choices—things like alcohol abuse, addiction, infidelity, domestic abuse, failed relationships, and estrangements.

But worst of all, many first responders feel shame because they know they need help, and they believe that asking for help is taboo in their profession.

Shame causes people to feel so bad about themselves and their circumstances that they will often lash out aggressively or withdraw completely from the people in their lives. They also turn on themselves. Feeling devalued and unworthy of love, acceptance, and connection, they exist in a vicious cycle of self-hatred, grief, anxiety, and depression. Shame causes isolation, separation, pain, and disconnection, and it prevents people from asking for help.

## They Mask and Numb

In an effort to ignore and avoid their pain, some first responders keep themselves distracted and/or sedated. Addictions range from sex to gambling, from alcoholism to prescription drug use, and everything in between.

They overeat, overcompensate, and overindulge. They become workaholics. They pretend to be someone they're not. They joke around, work out like crazy, drink like rock stars—anything to keep them from facing what's going on inside.

# They Sometimes Want to Die, and Sometimes They Do

Six of the nine first responders I interviewed confided in me that they have either contemplated suicide, wished they would die, imagined death as relief, believed the world would be better off without them, or wondered what it would be like if they didn't exist anymore.

That's 66.7 percent.

I can't prove this, but I'm going to venture to guess that this is a good representation of first responders nationwide, maybe even worldwide. If that's true, then we can safely say that nearly 70 percent of our first responders have thought about dying as a way to escape the pain and trauma of their work.

Let's all pause here for a few seconds and take that in.

Couple more seconds.

Are you processing this?!

These cultures have groomed individuals to be so averse to seeking help for mental and emotional issues that they sometimes imagine death as their only hope. For some, the thoughts are fleeting, without serious consideration of self-harm. They just find themselves thinking, "What if that semi swerved right now and killed me?" Or, "I wonder if my kids would be okay if I weren't here." For others, thoughts of death and dying become a preoccupation. Then there are those who have considered and contemplated suicide, and still others who have plans in place, but have not yet taken action to end their own lives.

And then there are those who have survived suicide attempts.

More firefighters and police officers die by suicide than in the line of duty, and this has been true for at least a couple of years. As of the writing of this book, approximately twenty military veterans die by suicide *every day*. And suicide is becoming more and more prevalent in all the other first-responder professions as well.

I hope each and every person who reads or hears the words in this section is as dumbfounded as I am as I type them. Our first responders—the people responsible for saving our lives—are so traumatized that they sometimes want to die.

And sometimes they do.

# Chapter 6

# SUICIDAL IDEATION

### Thoughts, Talk, Plans

Suicidal ideation means having thoughts about suicide or wanting to take one's own life. There are two primary types of suicidal ideation: passive and active.

Passive suicidal ideation means a person thinks about death and dying or wishes they would die, but doesn't have a plan in place to kill themself.

Active suicidal ideation is when a person has the intent to kill themself and has a plan to do so.

A few months ago, I participated in a train-the-trainer class for a first-responder wellness class called *Building Resilience and Surviving Secondary Trauma*. This class takes a pretty deep dive into first-responder mental and emotional health, as well as suicide.

The instructor told us that, when we suspect someone might be suicidal, it's not enough to ask if they are considering harming themselves, or any other limp-noodle version of this question. He taught us to ask the direct and pointed question, "Are you planning to kill yourself?" Then, if the person hesitates or answers with any version close to a yes, he instructed us to ask this very important follow-up question, "Do you have a plan?" If it's a yes, he warned, you must take immediate action.

Suicide has become a serious national epidemic and is prevalent throughout all first-responder professions. First responders, those who love them, and those, like me, who want desperately to help them, must become aware of the signs of suicidal ideation and be willing to take action if necessary.

What does it mean to take action? The possibilities are endless, and it depends on the circumstances. The only thing that's not okay is *inaction* if someone indicates they have a suicide plan. You can't walk away, shrug it off, or let it go and hope for the best. However, if a person in your life does complete suicide, in spite of all efforts to help and support them, you must never blame yourself for their death. Ultimately, we are each responsible for our own choices.

# THE COMMON PREDICTORS OF FIRST-RESPONDER SUICIDE

The following list of symptoms can be signs or indicators that the possibility of suicide exists, especially if multiple symptoms are concurrent, chronic, or repetitive.

- Chronic stress
- Depression
- Anxiety
- Anger
- Intense irritability
- Aggression
- Alcohol abuse/ alcoholism

- Drug use/addiction
- Hopelessness
- Isolation/withdrawal
- Suicidal ideation
- Talk of suicide

If you are experiencing multiple symptoms concurrently, do not hesitate to ask for help. Don't wait. Don't let your pride or fear get in the way. Reach out to someone and tell them you need help, then accept the help, and do whatever it takes to feel better and live better. Know that what you're experiencing is treatable; you can recover from this, no matter how bad you're feeling today. You *can* feel better and you can go on to live your best life.

Please, reach out right now.

Call a friend, call the National Suicide Prevention Lifeline, or text the Crisis Text Line.

---

National Suicide Prevention Lifeline:
1-800-273-8255

Crisis Text Line:
Text HOME to 741741

---

Part 3

# THE
# WISDOM

## Chapter 7

# MEDITATION AND MINDFULNESS

### What They Are and How They Can Help

I view meditation and mindfulness as brain training exercises. I say they are rooted in common sense and backed by science. This is how I approach these practices, and this is how I teach them.

---

**Meditation Disclaimer for Skeptics**

If you think meditation is not for you because it's weird, hippy-dippy, new-agey, or is only for Buddhists and monks, please set those preconceptions aside. Meditation is not necessarily connected with, or in opposition to, any spiritual philosophy or religion. It can be, but it can also be used as a secular brain training exercise for the purpose of stress relief and other benefits.

---

# What Is Meditation?

Here is a simple definition of meditation: a few minutes of uninterrupted silence each day.

Meditation is a practice or an exercise that brings your awareness into the present moment, and that is what we're going to focus on in this segment of the book—the importance of being able to bring your own attention into the present moment.

Now, when I say "silence" in the definition, I don't mean that everything is supposed to go completely silent around you and inside your head. What I mean is that you are not talking or watching television or interacting with anything that is overstimulating or requires you to mentally engage.

Some people like to listen to guided meditations or play soft music, white noise, or sounds of nature when they meditate, and that is fine.

Also, you do not have to silence your thoughts. That is impossible, and trying to do so is stressful. With practice and perseverance, you will learn what to do when thoughts occur, and over time you will notice the thoughts begin to settle and subside.

To me, meditation is the act of *being*. Some other good descriptions are observing, becoming familiar with, accepting, releasing, expanding, and allowing.

# What Is Mindfulness?

Here is a simple definition of mindfulness: awareness in the present moment without judgment.

Mindfulness is a state of being, a way of living. Mindfulness invites you to place your attention on the present moment in time and become aware of the self. When you are mindful, you are checked into the here and now and tuned into yourself.

One deep, slow, full breath can initiate mindfulness. As you inhale, you shift your attention from wherever it was to this breath. This brings your awareness into the present moment, because your inhale is taking place in the present moment in time, and if you are focused on it, you are focused in the present moment in time.

But how do you stay there?

You take another breath. You expand and deepen these breaths. You slow them down and hold your attention on them. You feel the oxygen coming into your body and observe what's happening internally as you breathe. You listen for the sound of your inhale and exhale. You do whatever works for you to hold your own attention on the breathing, and the self. It's all about observing and feeling.

Now that you have your own attention, enjoy how it feels. Continue breathing. Feel for any sensations that might be occurring in your body. Notice how your body feels. Observe what is happening right now. Focus on how your body feels in your seat. Notice the heaviness and density of your body, feel your rear end in the chair, feel your back against the seat, notice how your feet feel in your shoes or how your feet feel on the floor. These are all ways to practice mindfulness.

You can use mindfulness as an exercise, for distraction from stress and overwhelm. When you do, there is an immediate experience of relief, focus, and mental clarity.

You can also implement mindfulness throughout your day as a relaxation tool or a self-regulation skill. Practicing mindfulness helps you become more aware of your thoughts, feelings, and bodily sensations. If you wish to improve or change your mental or emotional state, you must first become aware of your *current* mental or emotional state. Mindfulness makes that possible.

If you aren't living mindfully, then you are probably living habitually or mindlessly, consistently doing the same things in the same way, repeating patterns and making the same choices and mistakes over and over again, day after day. Like many people, you are living on autopilot, in some form of survival mode.

### Without Judgment

What do I mean by "without judgment?" Practicing non-judgment in the present moment means that you avoid the typical, automatic tendency toward labeling, criticizing, categorizing, quantifying, qualifying, or complaining about what you are experiencing in the moment. Instead of *judging*, you practice *accepting*.

Let me give you an example.

Let's say you have a very important appointment. You leave a little late, you run into traffic, and then you see construction up ahead. Now you are going to be very late. What is your automatic response?

If you are a road-rage person, your automatic response is most likely anger, hostility, maybe even rage. You feel agitated, stressed, and anxious. If you pay attention, you can literally *feel* this in your body. As this occurs, your breathing might become shallow or labored, your heart rate begins to increase, and your blood pressure begins to rise. You grip the steering wheel tightly.

You clench your teeth. Your shoulders are tight and constricted. You ride bumpers and weave in and out of traffic. Mentally, you are raging against yourself, angry that you left late instead of leaving on time. Outwardly, you are raging against the other drivers, the traffic, and the stupid Department of Transportation that decided construction on the highway at this time of day was a good idea.

I might have gotten a little carried away there with my description, but for those of you who lean toward road rage, it's probably not much of an exaggeration.

Why is this reaction and behavior a big deal? Because each and every time you have an automatic mental, emotional, and physical reaction like this, you are creating stress in your own system. The labored or shallow breathing, racing heart, and elevated blood pressure are probably causing stress hormones such as adrenaline and cortisol to flood your system. You don't need me to tell you this and you don't need to do any research, because you can *feel* this happening in your body, if you are aware. And that's the key—awareness.

If you have a desire to learn how to modulate yourself when faced with a crisis (self-inflicted or otherwise), and you believe that self-regulation would be a helpful tool, the first thing you need to pay attention to is your own attention. Where is your focus? Where is your awareness? What are you thinking about, dwelling on, obsessing over? Practicing mindfulness can help you increase your awareness, and that is a powerful shift.

In this road-rage example, "without judgment" would mean you would not initiate a mental rant of judgment against yourself, the other drivers, or the construction. Instead of judging, you would accept the situation as it is. Because the situation *is* as it is. Your lack of acceptance of that fact only serves to create resistance to *what is* (what is actually occurring in this moment that is out of your control). Resisting *what is* means trying to *control the uncontrollable*. It is futile and, honestly, a bit insane.

*Awareness in the present moment without judgment* might go like this: "Okay. I left a little late, I'm in traffic, and I'm going to be late." (This is acceptance of *what is*.) Now, instead of *reacting* habitually with road rage, you make the empowering choice to *respond* to the situation in whatever way is appropriate. Do you need to make a phone call and let someone know you're going to be late? Do that. And then go about massaging your awareness into the present moment by breathing and using the techniques I'm going to teach you in this book. Why? Because of the *relief* you will feel and the *stress reduction* you will experience.

## What Is the Present Moment?

The present moment can also be called "now." It is this current moment in time. How do you know when you are focused in the present moment? When you are neither thinking about something from the past nor thinking about something in the future, that is when you are focused in the present moment.

### The Past

The past is any moment in time that came before this now moment. That can mean five minutes ago, twelve years ago, or when you were a child. It's all the same. It's all in the past. The important thing to note about the past is that it's *gone*. It no longer exists. The past only exists in your mind and in your memories. You can't go back. You can't redo or undo anything. You have no power in the past. All you can do is think about it. And yet, we tend to spend a lot of time and energy mentally dwelling in the past, don't we?

The problem with past-thinking is that it often makes us feel bad. It tends to bring with it unpleasant memories and images, and feelings of resentment, guilt, and regret. So thinking about the past can make us feel sad, depressed, and angry. If you are a person who leans toward past-thinking, you might also lean toward feeling depressed, low, or disempowered.

So, am I telling you that you should never think about the past? No. I'm asking you to begin to discern how past-thinking makes you feel. You can train yourself to recognize when past-thinking feels good, like a nostalgic, fond memory, and when it feels bad, like a disturbing memory of a dark time in your life. Then, when it feels bad, you can make the choice to bring your awareness out of the past and into the present.

Often, when I talk about this subject, people will ask, "What about the importance of learning lessons from the past? If I don't think back on what has occurred in the past, I might not learn the lesson." To that I say, take the lesson, but leave the story. The thing that causes us to feel *bad* when we mentally drift into the past is the habit of replaying the incident or memory over and over in our minds, or retelling the story of it over and over to anyone who will listen. Again, this becomes a matter of discernment. You must learn to recognize and identify how you're feeling.

When you are fully focused in the present moment, the past loses its power to make you feel bad. Here's an example. If you are watching a comedy on TV and you are fully present and paying attention to it, you feel pretty good. Why? Because your awareness is focused *in this now moment* on *what's right in front of you*. In that moment, you are not feeling bad about past events because you are not *focused* on them. But you won't always need something external, like TV, to distract you or hold your attention. You can learn to bring your own awareness into the present moment by focusing internally and holding your focus there, and you will experience the same outcome, with the added element of peace and empowerment.

Sound difficult, or maybe even impossible? Trust me, it isn't. It takes some work and practice to learn this skill because the past is a strong magnet, and it will pull your thoughts and attention back if you aren't vigilant. However, if you want to experience the liberating relief of letting the past go and enjoying the rewarding power of the present, you have the ability to train yourself to do so, using the power of meditation and mindfulness.

### The Future

The future, like the past, does not exist in this present moment. You can't *do* anything or *affect* anything in the future, because it isn't here yet. All you can do is *think* about it and worry. And *that's* the problem with future-thinking. We can't control the future with future-thinking, but we sure do spend a lot of time mentally focused there, don't we?

When you focus your thoughts into the future, you are typically worrying or practicing worst-case-scenario thinking or precautionary thinking. You are attempting to imagine all the bad things that might possibly happen so you can be prepared if they do. Being as prepared as possible for the future is one thing; obsessively worrying about future events you cannot possibly control until you're filled with fear and anxiety is quite another.

Preparedness is a necessity in first-responder professions, I will grant you that. Precautionary thinking is a part of the job. But do you find yourself practicing it all the time? Are there times and places in your personal life when you could let up on it a little? I am not asking you to *never* think ahead. I am simply suggesting that you begin to discern how future-thinking makes you feel—and how it makes the people in your personal life feel.

My husband always had a plan, and a Plan B, and honestly a plan for all twenty-six letters in the alphabet. He was prepared at all times for any catastrophe or tragedy that might occur. Part of this simply had to do with his make-up and personality. But he developed some of it as a result of the disorder and dysfunction he experienced in his life and as a cop. He felt preparedness and precautionary thinking were crucial in society and in the home, to avoid chaos.

David was so accustomed to using future-thinking as a precautionary tactic that he lost his ability to modulate it. He tried to apply preemptive "law and order" strategies at home that were well-intended, but a step too far. He was always looking around for what might go wrong. "Head on a swivel," as they say in law enforcement. This is known as hypervigilance, and it's very common among first responders. For first responders, and their families, it can conjure stress, fear, and anxiety.

Future-thinking always involves worry, worry causes fear, and fear creates anxiety. Therefore, future-thinking creates anxiety.

What's the antidote? Present-moment awareness. The act of consciously shifting your awareness out of the future and into this moment in time can ease the anxiety caused by worrying about the future. Present-moment awareness settles your attention into the here and now, and that brings relief.

So what about planning, you might ask? How can I make plans and set goals if I'm not supposed to think into the future?

I'm not asking you to avoid *ever* thinking about the future. I'm simply inviting you to begin practicing discernment when you find yourself future-focused. Notice how you feel. Is there tension or anxiety present in your body? Do you feel worried or fearful? If so, try using the tools I'm going to teach you in this book to bring your awareness into the present moment and experience the relief that's available to you.

## Why Meditate?

Meditation is an exercise that helps you focus your attention into the present moment. So essentially, practicing meditation is sort of like strengthening your attention muscle. With patience and repetition, this will become easier and easier, and soon you will discover the ability to consciously bring your awareness into the present moment any time you choose.

When you meditate, you sit still in a comfortable position, allow your muscles to relax, and breathe. As you sit, you observe your breathing, your thoughts, and how you are feeling. You surrender into the present moment. You enter into a state of *being*, not *doing*, not trying to force outcomes. Just being.

During meditation, if you notice thoughts that are unsettling or stressful, you have the option to either observe those thoughts without judgment, or gently shift your awareness away from the thoughts, to the sound, feeling, and rhythm of your breathing. Or you can observe how your body feels by noticing sensations and subtle vibrations that might be detectable. Any of these passive options will serve to hold your awareness in the present moment.

When you surrender into the present moment, the future does not exist, nor does the past. You are not thinking about the past, worrying about the future, or focusing on people and circumstances you cannot control. You are simply being, with yourself, in the moment.

The present moment has many gifts to offer and there are many benefits available to you when you practice meditation.

### Stress Reduction

Meditation is an evidence-based practice that helps you learn to manage and reduce your own stress, and I will discuss some of the scientific and empirical benefits later in this chapter. When you sit in meditation, you are still and quiet. You're breathing fully and deeply, which oxygenates your system. This assists in slowing down your heart rate, which can begin to lower your blood pressure. Your muscles begin to relax. Instead of going, doing, and thinking, you are slowing down. You are discovering how it feels to simply *be*. You are disengaging from all activity. You are giving yourself a beautiful gift of a few minutes of stillness in which all the functions of the brain and body have an opportunity to settle, calm, and regulate.

### Emotional Regulation, Self-Regulation

Emotional regulation and self-regulation become like superpowers once you get the hang of them. When you practice meditation and mindfulness, you become familiar with the power of observation. You learn to pull your awareness into the present moment and shift your attention to self. Then you observe. You just breathe, feel, and observe.

Before you can regulate your emotions, you have to feel them, observe them, and become familiar with them. Once you get comfortable with the practice of observing, you can learn to identify emotions that aren't serving you well and, instead of being flooded by them, you can develop the ability to modulate or regulate them.

Can you imagine having the power and ability to modulate your own emotions when you choose to? Think of instances both professionally and personally in which this might be a powerful skill to possess.

Disclaimer: I am not suggesting that anyone ignore, override, or deny emotions. If, in this process of discovery, you find you have difficult emotions that continue to adversely impact you and those around you, please seek professional help.

What I am addressing is our ability to evolve from habitual, reactionary individuals to more balanced beings by becoming familiar with and learning to balance the emotions that hold us back. A person who is habitually quick to anger can learn to observe and feel the anger, identify its origin, decipher whether or not it is appropriate in the moment, and modulate it when desired.

Here is a great example. A friend of mine, who was in the military and is now a police officer, tells the story of a time, before he discovered meditation and stepped onto a healing path, when he expressed hostility toward his then-five-year-old son. The little boy knocked over a glass of milk and began to cry. My friend reacted harshly, yelling at his son and making him cry harder. Looking back, my friend realizes he wasn't angry at the boy for spilling the milk, he was angry at him for crying. He had come to view any emotion other than anger as "soft." Anger had become my friend's primary emotion, and it was habitual. It was ruling him and ruining his relationships.

When my friend tells this story, you can see the emotion on his face and in his eyes. But, through a process of healing, using meditation as his primary tool, he has developed the ability to recognize and identify his emotions, and regulate them when he chooses to. He has *become familiar with* his emotions through meditation. (Refer back to my definition of meditation and the list of descriptions I included.)

At home, self-regulation will help you become a more effective communicator. Plus, you will be setting a powerful example for anyone you live with, especially children. This skill can definitely help you develop healthier relationships.

The same thing applies on the job. Take a moment to think about areas of your professional life that could be enhanced by developing this skill. Think of circumstances and interactions with others that might be enhanced or defused when you start to apply emotional regulation, or self-regulation.

### Personal Empowerment

Personal empowerment means you feel more in charge of your own life. Learning to bring your own awareness into the present moment and apply emotional regulation empowers you to respond to people and situations instead of reacting. That, my friends, is empowering.

Do you ever feel like an old, tattered flag being whipped around in the wind? Do you ever feel as though you have very little power in your own life? Would you like to feel more empowered? More in charge? Would you like to possess the life-enhancing skill of response, as opposed to reactivity? Imagine how much more empowered you will feel.

## Inner Peace

Now, before you roll your eyes at this term, hear me out. I'm not talking about some hippie lovefest where we all join hands and sing and channel our inner Gandhi. Inner peace is simply the opposite of inner chaos.

We all know what inner mental and emotional chaos feels like. We know that overthinking and an overactive mind contributes to stress and anxiety. And we've all experienced emotional chaos, when our feelings seem to take over and flood us, resulting in unhealthy reactions to people and circumstances.

What I am suggesting is an undoing of that, a settling of mental activity and emotional upheaval that brings about quieting and a calm feeling inside: inner peace.

## Meditation Cultivates Mindfulness

I like to say that meditation is to mindfulness as exercise is to physical fitness.

If you want to achieve better overall physical fitness, you know you have to exercise. There's just no way around it. You also know you have to exercise regularly. Sure, you could go to the gym right now, get in a good workout, and feel great! Endorphins would kick in, and you would leave the gym with an elevated feeling. But you won't wake up tomorrow morning physically fit. Achieving physical fitness takes time, repetition, and regularity.

Similarly, if you want to begin to experience more mindfulness in your life, meditation is a great exercise to help you achieve that goal. Mindfulness is a way of life, a state of being. When you are mindful, you are more present in your own life. More checked-in, tapped-in and tuned-in to yourself and the present moment. Less distracted. Less reactive.

Remember, earlier I said the practice of meditation brings your awareness into the present moment? It's like flexing your present-moment awareness muscle. When you sit in a few minutes of meditation each day, you are practicing the skill of bringing your attention into the present moment. Over time, you will be able to call upon that skill in any given moment. Choosing to pull yourself consciously into the present moment will become second nature to you.

So, if you want to experience more presence in your life, if you want mindfulness to weave itself into the tapestry of your life, practice meditation. Meditation cultivates mindfulness.

## My Approach to Meditation

I view meditation as a brain training exercise. Initially, sitting in stillness and silence while doing nothing but breathing and being might feel counterintuitive to you. This is normal. When you sit, especially in the beginning, you might feel restless, fidgety, bored, anxious, or a multitude of other things. But with some practice, you can train your brain (and body) to allow the stillness and embrace the silence.

## Brain Training Exercise

Training your brain to sit and stay is kind of like training a puppy. When you first get a puppy, it will not understand the command to sit and stay. It will be wriggly and jumpy and dart all over the place. But with some patience, practice, and repetition, you can train that puppy to do what you are asking it to do.

The same goes for your brain. With some commitment and dedication, you can train your brain out of automatic, habitual thinking and activity. At first, the brain might become very active. It might frantically remind you that you have things to do and things to worry about and to-do lists to make and attack. It will throw all its habitual worries, cares, concerns, and random thoughts at you.

But you will gently show your brain who's in charge. By learning some of the tips and tools that I'm going to share with you in this book, you can train your brain to allow the stillness and silence that can reap so many positive benefits.

This really is the biggest hurdle for most people in the beginning, but don't worry! I'm going to teach you some skills you can apply that will force your brain to comply and yield to the inactivity that is so very beneficial to your entire system.

## Rooted in Common Sense

We live in a society in which action, going, doing, and thinking are prevalent, praised, and valued. We receive validation for our busyness, and we tend to value busy people above what we might consider lazy people. Being skilled in the act of doing nothing is not usually high on the list of one's accomplishments. But I feel we should all rethink that.

I believe people used to innately understand the importance of doing nothing for a few minutes each day. Did you know that people used to sit on their front porches and watch the world go by? When I was a kid, I spent a lot of time with my grandparents. I remember in the evening, after dinner, they would usually just sit for a while. If the weather was nice, they would sit outside on their patio. They would not automatically turn on a radio or television. They would just sit.

In modern times, if we say we are going to relax, that usually means we sit on a couch in front of a television, we have a remote control, a smartphone, and maybe a laptop or tablet. That might feel relaxing, but you are still actively engaged mentally, visually, and auditorily. I'm encouraging you to learn to *disengage* from all of that and simply learn to sit quietly with yourself.

When you meditate, that's exactly what you do. You sit for a few minutes and disengage—from everything. You can listen to a guided meditation, some soft music, white noise, or the sounds of nature in the background while you sit, but the practice requires you to disengage from your physical environment, from devices, and from other people.

Doing so gives your brain and body a chance to settle, to reset and recalibrate. In other words, there is nothing for you to do during meditation. You're not trying to force an outcome. All the benefits that are available to you through meditation will happen naturally; you just have to allow for that possibility.

Doesn't it seem like good old-fashioned common sense that this might be good for you?

## Backed by Science

Meditation and mindfulness have made their way into the mainstream. There have been thousands of scientific papers written on the evidence-based health benefits of meditation. Some of those benefits include:

- Lower blood pressure
- Reduced anxiety
- Alleviated depression

- Diminished sleep problems
- Enhanced immune system
- Improved brain function

While more studies are needed and research is ongoing, there's compelling data to support meditation as a viable tool to improve mental, emotional, and physical health.

### *Lower Blood Pressure*

It is well-documented that stress contributes to high blood pressure, and there are numerous studies linking meditation to lower blood pressure. Practically speaking, when you sit in meditation and focus on deep, slow breathing, your entire body begins to relax. This relaxation helps calm and reduce the symptoms of stress, which can lead to lower blood pressure, especially when meditation is practiced regularly.

### *Reduced Anxiety*

Anxiety is an emotional state precipitated by perceived threats, worry, and fear of the unknown and uncontrollable. Meditation has been shown to help regulate brain function and balance body chemistry, which can help reduce the symptoms of anxiety.

### *Alleviated Depression*

Depression is a mood disorder that is marked by persistent feelings of sadness, emptiness, hopelessness, pessimism, irritability, and fatigue. Meditation has been linked to mental, emotional, and even physical regulation and balancing, which can help reduce the symptoms of depression.

### *Diminished Sleep Problems*

Meditation is a great sleep aid, largely because it raises levels of melatonin in the body. But those who meditate also have other advantages in getting a good night's sleep. The breathing and relaxation techniques used in meditation, paired with the ability to quiet the mind, can help promote better sleep.

### *Enhanced Immune System*

Chronic stress keeps the body in a state of detrimental activation, which increases wear and tear on biological systems. Meditation offers rest and deep relaxation to help the body come into balance, function optimally, protect itself against viruses and other infections, and repair existing damage.

### *Improved Brain Function*

Of particular interest to me, in my work with first responders, is the research showing deactivation and decreased gray matter in the part of the brain called the amygdala. The amygdala plays a key role in the processing of emotions and controls the stress response, also known as the fight or flight response.

When the stress response is turned on, the body releases stress hormones such as cortisol into the system. High levels of cortisol have been linked to moderate and severe health problems. Studies show that first responders tend to have high levels of cortisol due to hyperactivity in the amygdala, and that often the amygdala is enlarged in the brains of first responders.

Research indicates that meditation rewires, restructures, and physically changes the brain. Studies demonstrate that meditation causes decreased activation and decreased gray matter in the areas of the brain associated with stress, while increasing activation in the areas associated with a positive mental attitude, self-awareness, decision-making, and compassion.

For more on this, please refer to Harvard neuroscientist Dr. Sarah Lazar's studies from 2005 and 2011 on how meditation affects the brain. Or you can read the 2011 article *Eight Weeks to a Better Brain*, published by the *Harvard Gazette* online, which highlights Dr. Lazar's work.

In general, neuroscience is telling us that intentional activation and deactivation of certain areas of the brain initiates neuroplasticity (the brain's ability to adapt and change), and that meditation is one tool we can use to promote neuroplasticity, thereby improving brain function.

If you are interested in learning more about the benefits of meditation, all you have to do is search "meditation articles" on your computer and start reading!

## Why Practice Mindfulness?

There are two aspects to mindful awareness that we talk about in my classes, and I want to cover these in some depth here. When you begin practicing mindfulness, it is important to understand

The Mindfulness for Warriors Handbook

the process and the goal. The two aspects of awareness are self-awareness and present-moment awareness.

## Present-Moment Awareness

I like to initiate this conversation by talking to people about the power of the present moment in time. In order to become familiar with the present moment, you first have to realize that the present moment is now. Right now. This exact moment in time. It's also important to remember that the time is always *now*.

You might look at your watch and see that it is 4:11 p.m. Central Standard Time. But the actual time is *now*. Take a moment to think about this. *Now* is the only moment in time that ever actually exists, the only moment in time in which you have any power to do anything. The past is gone, and the future isn't here yet.

## Self-Awareness

I cannot emphasize the importance of self-awareness enough. Tuning into one's self and becoming familiar with how one is doing and feeling mentally, emotionally, and physically is a powerful process. Unfortunately, in our modern society, we have been trained into external focus. From an early age, we are taught to mentally override pain and discomfort. We are encouraged to put other people ahead of ourselves and to ignore our own desires, discomfort, concerns, and even pain.

I am suggesting that it's time for us to become a little more self-centered, in a healthy way, by becoming *centered in self*. Becoming more aware of one's own state of being and needs is healthfully selfish, in my opinion. It will not diminish your ability to take care of others and offer yourself in service to the greater good. The opposite is actually true.

There is a reason why flight attendants tell us to secure our own oxygen mask before we help anybody else, even our own children. I remember being a young mother, flying with my infant daughter for the first time. When I heard the flight attendant give those instructions I thought, no way. There is absolutely no way I am going to take care of myself first.

Fast-forward a few years into mothering and a couple of kids later. Not only did I understand the practical application of that instruction, the metaphor became glaringly apparent. In trying to be a good mom, I got in the habit of putting everything and everyone ahead of myself. Therefore, after several years, I began to feel depleted and resentful.

Does this sound familiar? Do you ever feel underappreciated, overworked, and used-up? Do you take good care of yourself and tend to your own needs? Or do you give everything away, neglecting yourself in an effort to take care of everything and everyone else?

Several years ago, I was working with a private client. She was going through a very stressful time in her life, and she wanted to learn how to meditate. She was in the middle of a divorce, moving out of the home she had lived in for twenty years, and she had taken a new position with a new company. Toward the end of her session, we did a meditation together. As we came out of the meditation, I noticed she was crying. She shared with me that, during the meditation, once she got still and quiet, her knee started hurting very badly. She went on to explain that this was nothing new. She had a bad knee that would eventually require surgery, but she was so stressed and busy that she simply had not taken the time to address it.

Then she said to me, I'm not crying because my knee hurts. My knee always hurts, I just mentally override it and push through. I'm crying because, during the meditation, I realized I am never still, I am never quiet, and I don't take care of myself.

I could tell this was an important epiphany for her. Before she left, she vowed to make that doctor's appointment she had been putting off and committed to taking better care of herself.

If you desire to make any improvements or changes in your life, regarding your health, happiness, relationships, finances, or anything else, it is imperative that you become familiar with yourself and what's going on within you—your thoughts, feelings, needs, and desires. You must practice self-awareness.

This is where mindfulness comes in. Mindfulness leaves the past, stays out of the future, focuses in the present moment, and is aware of self. Now, let's learn how to begin working with these powerful new concepts.

# Chapter 8

# BREATH: THE BODY'S NATURAL STRESS RELIEVER

"Breath is the bridge which connects life
to consciousness, which unites your body
to your thoughts."

**—Thich Nhat Hanh**

We humans have an amazing built-in mechanism for self-regulation, and it is the breath. What a gift!

In every class I teach, I repeat over and over: *the breath is the body's natural stress reliever.* I want it to sink in. I feel like, even if people don't fully embrace meditation or begin practicing mindfulness, if they can just start remembering to breathe *on purpose*, they will begin to know relief.

I encourage my students to take breathing breaks during the day. We discuss ways they can start applying mini or micro practices throughout each day to reduce stress and feel better, and breathing is the primary practice.

Deepening and regulating the breath can help slow down the heart rate and begin lowering blood pressure. Muscles begin to relax. This purposeful or conscious breathing brings almost immediate relief from stress, agitation, and anxiety, and can initiate mental clarity when one is experiencing mental overwhelm.

## Breathing into the Present Moment

If you are stressed, anxious, fearful, overwhelmed, etc., you are most likely not focused here and now. You are probably mentally elsewhere, thinking about the past, the future, or something or someone you can't control.

When you breathe deeply, slowly, and purposefully, and you focus your attention on this breathing by observing it, feeling it, and/or listening to it, you are simultaneously distracting yourself from the thoughts, distractions, worries, fears, confusion, or other mental chaos that's causing you to feel stressed.

In other words, paying attention to your breathing, while focusing on slowing it down and deepening it, brings your awareness fully into the present moment. Your breathing is happening *here* and *now*. So, when you pay attention to your breathing, your awareness is focused *here and now*, otherwise known as the present moment.

The simple act of breathing yourself into the present moment can bring great relief from stress, worry, overthinking, and other mental stressors.

# Breathe like a Baby

We live in a society of shallow breathers who are rarely focused in the present moment. When we are stressed, the breath is the first thing to go. Our breath becomes shallow, choppy, labored, or we might even hold our breath. When this occurs, we are not functioning optimally. Shallow breathing prevents full oxygenation of the system, which can cause tension, stress, and anxiety. The body and brain *need* oxygen to function properly. Shallow breathing limits the delivery of oxygen to the system and can even trigger the sympathetic nervous system, which activates the fight or flight response.

To counteract this, we need to learn to breathe like a baby.

Have you ever noticed an infant lying on its back in a crib? Babies naturally breathe fully. If you watch, you'll notice their entire belly and abdomen fully expand with each breath and contract with each exhale. This is known as diaphragmatic breathing. Diaphragmatic breathing occurs when we use the diaphragm to breathe. The diaphragm is a muscle located below the lungs that controls respiration.

We all start out, as infants, breathing fully and deeply, but over time, stress, anxiety, and other factors affect our breathing, converting us from deep breathers to shallow breathers. Diaphragmatic breathing, or "belly breathing," as I call it in my classes, serves many purposes, not the least of which is, it *feels good*. I call it belly breathing because the way to know you're doing it right is to make sure your belly is expanding, and honestly, I just think it's easier for most people to remember.

Babies breathe fully, the way humans *should* breathe, because babies haven't yet developed the habits of worrying, regretting, ruminating, overthinking, and obsessing. These mental distractions keep adult human beings (and some children) in a constant state of stress, which can lead to shallow breathing.

Learning how to use diaphragmatic breathing, or belly breathing, can improve your health, primarily by improving oxygenation and reducing stress. When you're stressed, your body uses a lot of its resources to deal with the stress. Reduce that stress, and your body can use those freed-up resources to do what it was created to do: get and keep you in balance, also known as homeostasis.

## How to Get Started

Let's give belly breathing a try. You can practice sitting up or lying on your back.

- Start by placing one hand on your belly, and the other hand on your upper chest.

- Breathe slowly in through your nose, pulling air all the way down into your belly.

- The inhale should be full and deep, and the hand on your belly should be moving as your belly expands.

- Exhale completely through your nose (or through your mouth if breathing through the nose is uncomfortable for you), but keep the exhale slow and steady.

- Slow down and extend or elongate the exhale for added stress relief.

- As you breathe, observe the expansion of your belly, abdomen, and chest, and notice how you feel.

- Repeat for several breaths.

There are a lot of breathing techniques that can help you reduce stress. You can explore some of these by doing a quick search on your computer. The important thing is to breathe fully and oxygenate your body!

## Breathing as a Mindful Practice

One deep, slow, purposeful breath is all you need to initiate mindfulness. It really is that simple. Focus on slowing the breathing down, and on long, full inhales and exhales. As you breathe, allow your attention to settle on the sound, feeling, and rhythm of the breaths. Observe. Feel. Stay with it. This alone is a mindful practice.

# Chapter 9

# LEARN TO PAUSE: MINDFULNESS TRAINING

## Conscious Breathing and Self-Coaching

The core of my current work is the four-hour block of mindfulness training I have designed as an introduction—a starting place for first responders and others who might be new to meditation and mindfulness.

In that class, I offer some super simple strategies for initiating mindfulness throughout the day, and I want to share some of those with you. To keep it doable, I encourage mini or micro (short, quick) practices that people can easily drop into their day.

The first step to remembering to initiate mindfulness throughout your day is to begin to analyze yourself periodically to determine how you're feeling. Next, you will need to remember and apply some strategies for dealing with stressful feelings when they arise.

The two main strategies I suggest are conscious breathing and self-coaching.

# Conscious Breathing

Remember, the breath is the body's natural stress reliever. Here are three quick and easy breathing techniques to try. Find one that works for you, and begin using it periodically throughout your day, any time you feel yourself getting tense, stressed, or anxious.

## Belly Breathing

The basics: You're going to inhale fully and deeply (through your nose as long as that's comfortable for you), making sure you're pulling the air all the way down, causing your belly to expand, then exhale slowly through your nose. This breathing should be slow, deep, and steady. Focus on slowing down and extending the exhale for added stress relief. Repeat until you feel an improvement, or for as long as you'd like.

See Chapter 8 for more tips on belly breathing.

## Breath Counting

If you need something to focus on while you breathe and work to settle your nervous system, try counting your breaths as you breathe.

The basics: You're going to begin taking slow, deep breaths, in and out through your nose, unless breathing through the nose is uncomfortable for you, in which case just breathe comfortably. As you breathe, count from one to four, over and over. Count a slow 1-2-3-4 on your inhale, and a slow 1-2-3-4 as you exhale.

Match the counting to your breathing, at your own pace, and repeat several times.

## 4-7-8 Breathing

This breathing technique will calm your nervous system and help you feel less stressed. Not everybody likes this exercise, but if it feels good to you, you can use it any time to relieve stress and tension.

The basics: You're going to inhale through your nose, then hold your breath, then exhale through your mouth, making a loud *whoosh* sound as you do.

Close your mouth and inhale quietly and deeply through your nose to a mental count of four. Hold your breath and mentally count to seven. Exhale completely through your mouth, making a *whoosh* sound as you mentally count to eight. This is one breath. Repeat this cycle three to four more times.

# Self-Coaching

To complement your new breathing techniques, here are a couple of easy-to-remember self-coaching strategies to help you practice mindfulness throughout your day. I call these the Three Qs and The Three Bs.

## The Three Qs

Here are three quick questions to ask yourself when you feel stressed, flooded, or overwhelmed:

1. Am I present?
2. What time is it?

3. Where am I?

Refer back to Chapter 7 and the discussion about present-moment awareness. Remember, we talked about how the present moment exists here and now and the fact that the time, no matter what the clock says, is always *now*.

Any time in the day you feel stress creeping up on you, pause, start taking deep, slow breaths, and ask yourself these three questions. And answer them, one by one!

The purpose of this exercise is to quickly snap you into the present moment—the only moment there ever really is.

## The Three Bs

A self-coaching tool and a mindful practice.

1. Breathe
2. Body
3. Be

I share The Three Bs with people all the time. The Three Bs initiate mindfulness, and they are also the first three steps of Pause15 Meditation, which we will learn about in the next chapter.

### *Breathe*

Begin taking deep, slow breaths. Start with some belly breaths to oxygenate your system. Focus on your breathing, feel the breaths enter your body, observe how they feel. Follow the breaths on the rise and fall.

### Body

As you continue to breathe, focus your awareness on your body. Notice how the breath feels coming in and exiting. Feel for any sensations you detect anywhere in your body. If you're sitting, feel your body against the chair. Notice the weight and density of your body. If you're standing, feel your feet on the floor. Sitting or standing, notice how your feet feel in your shoes. Wiggle your toes. Whatever it means for you to become aware of your body, do that. And just keep breathing.

### Be

Now, just be with this. Continue breathing. Gently hold your awareness on how the breath feels in your body, and how your body feels in this moment. If your mind begins to wander, you get distracted, or the stress persists, try taking another deep, slow breath, and allowing that breath to redirect you to the awareness of your breathing and your body.

# Chapter 10

# PAUSE15 MEDITATION

## Three Steps, Four Techniques, Fifteen Minutes a Day

Pause15 Meditation is a flexible meditation practice that caters to the individual. It's really a conglomeration of several different meditation techniques that I've put together over the years to try to reach beginners and entice people who are new to the idea of meditation.

Why do I call it Pause15? Because when I was starting out, the research showed that, in as little as fifteen minutes a day, you can reap all the benefits available from meditation. So I based my programs on fifteen-minute meditations.

My mission with this entire endeavor is to demystify meditation for people. My mission with Pause First is to normalize meditation and mindfulness in first-responder communities. So I keep it simple, and I offer flexibility within each technique I teach.

For example, if someone in a class says they can't possibly sit still and meditate for fifteen minutes, I ask them what they think they *can* do. Two minutes? Maybe three? Then I tell them to start there and meditate for a couple of minutes each day, but make sure they are doing it with discipline and commitment. I assure them they will realize one day that they are ready to add a minute, and I encourage them to keep adding a minute or two every so often, until they can sit for the full fifteen minutes!

There are many different meditation techniques out there, and I don't believe there is one perfect technique or one "right" way to meditate. We are all built very differently. We have different personalities, different lifestyles, and our brains operate differently. The best way to find a meditation practice that will work for you and is sustainable is to experiment and practice.

What I'm offering is an introduction, a starting point. If the concepts in this book appeal to you, and intellectually you connect with this information, but the meditation techniques I share don't appeal to you, don't give up! Take a class, find a book, download an app, do a Google search, or poke around on YouTube! I promise, you'll find something you connect with. There's so much to choose from!

## The Three Steps of Pause15 Meditation

### The Three Bs

1. Breathe
2. Body
3. Be

To start a meditation, use the same three steps you use to initiate mindfulness, The Three Bs—only, when you are meditating, they change slightly. You begin with breathing, but the second step becomes a *body scan*. We use the body scan to release tension and promote relaxation.

### Breathe

Begin taking deep, slow breaths. Start with some belly breaths to oxygenate your system. Focus on your breathing, feel the breaths enter your body, observe how they feel. Follow the breaths on the rise and fall.

### Body

This step becomes a body scan for relaxation. As you continue to breathe, focus your awareness on the top of your head and then, mentally scanning your way downward, imagine each part of your body relaxing and releasing tension as you mentally move all the way down your body to your feet.

Start by imagining your scalp releasing tension, then your forehead, your eyes, your cheeks, and your mouth. Keep breathing. Relax your neck, shoulders, and back...your chest, arms, hands, and fingers...your belly, hips, legs, feet, and toes. Just keep breathing as you mentally focus briefly on each of these areas and release tension.

### Be

Now, just be. This is meditation. During this phase of the meditation, you might need something to focus on to help you stay anchored in the meditation. Read through the four techniques in the next section and find one that feels comfortable to you.

Or simply try using your breathing as your anchor. Gently focus your awareness on your breathing throughout the entire meditation. When you get distracted or your mind begins to wander, try taking a nice deep, slow breath, and allow that breath to redirect you to your breathing.

Follow the breath on the rise and the fall. Notice how it feels coming into and leaving your body. Just follow the breath.

This part of the meditation is the actual meditation. But all three steps count toward your fifteen minutes. I recommend spending about five minutes on the breathing and body scan and then about ten minutes just being.

## Being

B Number Three really trips some people up. I totally understand, because sitting and doing nothing is counterintuitive to almost all of us.

But please take a moment to consider this. You are a human being, not a human doing. Being is your natural state. Imagine back to your first days of life, when you would lie in a crib all peaceful and innocent. First of all, you were *breathing deeply*, because babies do that. Also, you weren't worrying or fretting or overthinking like adults do. You were just a little being, *being*.

What I'm asking you to explore in meditation is that same state of being. You don't have to recreate it; you just have to get back in touch with it. You have grown so accustomed to going, doing, hustling, and forcing outcomes, you've lost touch with the concept of being. However, if you can slowly begin to train yourself into that state, all the evidence-based benefits that are available to your brain and body will happen naturally.

There is nothing for you to do, except ease yourself into a state of being, and you do that by simply allowing it to happen. You set the stage by breathing, settling into present-moment awareness, focusing on self, and allowing the process to occur naturally and organically.

In the state of being, your brain activity improves, your body chemistry begins to balance, your nervous system relaxes, and you begin to experience relief and clarity. So many wonderful things are possible for human beings when we allow ourselves to simply be.

Disclaimer: This process is challenging for most people. It takes time, practice, and perseverance, and you must trust the process. But it is achievable. Go easy on yourself; approach meditation as a marathon, not a sprint, and you will get the hang of it. You will begin to recognize that feeling of being, and you will come to crave it.

Your body, your system, is built for balance. Your body was created to get and keep you in homeostasis—in balance. You can't force this to happen, but you can allow it to. In meditation, instead of doing, you are allowing.

## Mental Chatter

To all of you Type-A personalities and perfectionists, and everyone else who might let a very active brain prevent them from trying meditation, please note the following:

> The goal of meditation is not to control your thoughts.
> It's to stop them from controlling you.

A common misperception about meditation is that you are supposed to sit in complete silence and stop or turn off your thoughts. Let me dispel that misperception right now.

Not only is stopping your thoughts not a requirement of meditation, it is, in fact, an impossibility. You do not have the ability to turn off your thoughts. There is a nonstop monologue going on in the back of your mind at all times. This consistent and persistent stream of mental analyzing, thinking, list-making, judging, labeling, and commenting happens without your conscious consent. We all have that mental chatter going on.

So the mental chatter will not automatically quiet down when you decide you want to meditate. The brain is habitual, and the chatter might be persistent in the beginning.

When this occurs, you can mentally say something like, "These words are the wind and my mind is a screen. I will let these words blow right through my mind."

Or you can think, "These words are the wind and my mind is a tree."

Using imagery like this might help you relax and disengage from habitual thinking and mental chatter.

Another trick you can try is naming or labeling your thoughts and then letting them go. Let's say you ease into a meditation and you are breathing and relaxing when a worrisome thought pops in. You can mentally say to yourself, "Oh, I recognize that, that is fear, but I don't wish to engage with it right now."

Then choose to let that thought go. Maybe you can imagine it floating away, or imagine putting it in a box and setting it to the side to be dealt with later. If you need to, you can develop little tricks like this which can free you up to continue breathing and relaxing.

With time and practice, you will see that, by applying a few of these tips, you can learn to experience the calm, quiet, and peace that's available in meditation. That mental chatter and those persistent thoughts will give up and float away eventually.

Remember, earlier I said you will need to train your brain to succumb to stillness and silence. If you can view this as an exercise or a practice and learn to relax through the difficult moments, you will also experience the serene moments. Just keep trying and be patient with yourself.

Disclaimer: Meditation is not always quiet and peaceful. It is important to allow meditation to be whatever it is. Sometimes you might feel fidgety and unsettled. Emotions might arise. Just try your best to ride those waves and sit through whatever happens. However, if you are extremely anxious, are experiencing panic attacks, or if meditation is a trauma trigger for you, *please seek professional help immediately.*

## The Four Techniques of Pause15 Meditation

1. Basic Daily Meditation
2. Breath Awareness Meditation
3. Counting Breaths Meditation
4. Mantra Meditation

Each meditation begins with The Three Bs. As you transition into step three (be), choose one of the techniques below to practice during the remainder of the meditation.

## Basic Daily Meditation

Simply close your eyes, breathe, relax your body, and allow yourself to be. Notice your breath. Breathe, feel, and observe. Observe thoughts instead of engaging with them. Allow whatever happens to happen.

## Breath Awareness Meditation

Focus on your breathing throughout the meditation to reduce distraction. When your mind wanders, take a nice deep breath and allow this breath to gently redirect you back to your breathing and the meditation. Follow the rhythm of your breath, feel the expansion of the breath, hear the breath...whatever it means to you to focus on your breathing. Use the breath to anchor you in the meditation.

## Counting Breaths Meditation

If you need something a little more tangible to help you stay connected with the meditation, try counting your breaths as you meditate. This one is good for very active minds. Count a slow 1-2-3-4 on your inhale, and a slow 1-2-3-4 as you exhale. Match your breathing to the counting. When your mind wanders, gently return to the counting. Count at your own pace as your breath gently ebbs and flows.

## Mantra Meditation

A mantra is a word or phrase you repeat mentally as you meditate. A mantra can help you stay anchored in the meditation. Try mentally repeating a calming word or phrase to prevent your mind from wandering. You can try using the word *relax*, by repeating the word over and over, at your own pace, as you meditate. Or you can try repeating the phrase *just be*. As you breathe, repeat *just* on the inhale, and *be* on the exhale. Mentally repeat your chosen word or phrase, over and over, as you breathe, relax, and be.

## Meditation FAQs

### What If I Fall Asleep?

It is common, especially when you're new to meditation, to fall asleep. Always meditate sitting up, and if you fall asleep, consider it much-needed rest. With practice, you'll benefit from the deep, rejuvenating rest meditation offers without nodding off.

### I Can't Turn Off My Mind! How Do I Stop the Thoughts?

This is the number-one complaint, and the primary reason people give up. Don't give up! Stick with it. Breathe, relax, and focus on neutrality—on being the observer of thoughts that pop in, without engaging. In time, the thoughts will slow down and your mind will become quiet.

### The Deep Breathing Is Uncomfortable, It Makes Me Anxious

Most of us are shallow breathers, so it might feel strange to breathe deeply, at first. Don't get hung up on the breathing. If it's distracting, just take a few deep breaths to get started, and then breathe naturally.

### Is It Better to Meditate Longer?

Research shows you benefit from meditating for as little as fifteen minutes per day. You can certainly meditate longer, but fifteen minutes or so every day is a sufficient length of time for most people.

### What Should I Do If I Get Interrupted While I'm Meditating?

There are no hard and fast rules. I recommend fifteen to twenty uninterrupted minutes. If there's a brief interruption, just settle back in and continue.

### Am I Supposed to Sit Motionless the Entire Time I'm Meditating?

No, if you become uncomfortable, you can shift around until you're comfortable. If you have an itch, scratch it. Just be as relaxed as possible.

### How Will I Know When My Fifteen Minutes Is Up?

You can sit near a clock and take an occasional peek, or set a soft, quiet alarm on your cell phone.

### Can I Meditate Lying Down?

I recommend sitting up, because lying down signals your body to sleep.

### What Is the Best Time of Day to Meditate?

The time of day when you meditate depends on your preferences and schedule. If you're not a morning person, trying to meditate in the morning might not be optimal. Choose a time of day that's right for you.

### Should I Meditate at the Same Time Every Day?

Creating a routine and establishing meditation as a regular daily practice is a great idea and will help you stick with it. But Plan B would be to fit it in once every day, as your schedule allows.

### How Do I Know If I'm Actually Meditating?

Consider it meditation, no matter what occurs in the fifteen to twenty minutes you devote to sitting and breathing in stillness, peace, and quiet.

### Is Meditation Good for Children?

Meditation is good for every single human being that walks this planet, with very few exceptions.

### Should I Meditate to Music, White Noise, or in Silence?

This is personal preference. Try different methods and techniques until you find one that works best for you. Or mix it up!

### Can I Count Cycling or Gardening as a Meditation?

While these activities might be relaxing and help you clear your mind, you are still engaged. You have to be in order to perform the activity. I really believe every single person on the planet should sit in uninterrupted silence for a few minutes each day and practice the art of simply being.

## Starting a Meditation Practice

You now know everything you need to know to begin meditating. I encourage you to seek out more information, do some research, get an app on your phone, or take a local class. But honestly, the best way to learn more about meditation is to do it! You can read every book ever written, listen to podcasts and scan the internet for information, but you won't discover nearly as much about meditation as you will by meditating.

Good luck, and let me know if I can help!

# Afterword

Dear Warrior,

I just realized these are the final words I will ever add to this book. It's been fun, emotional, and interesting to revisit the original book, add to it, include Keith's story, and enhance the resource section. Simultaneously, I've been working on my next book, *Wellness Warrior Style*, which I am excited to bring into the world soon.

In the meantime, I would love to hear from you if you have feedback or opinions you'd like to share. Input from readers helps me deliver better content, create more meaningful curriculum, and write the books people need and want to read.

I will provide my contact information and all the ways you can connect with me on the next page. Thank you for reading this book and thank you for your contribution to society. Please take good care of yourself. You deserve to live and retire healthfully.

With kind regards,
Kim

## Contact Info & Socials

*Kim Colegrove*

**Pause First Academy**

- Email: kimcolegrove@pausefirst.com

- Website: www.pausefirst.com

- Subscribe to my newsletter: www.pausefirst.com/contact

- Online Academy: www.academy.pausefirst.com

- LinkedIn: www.linkedin.com/in/kimcolegrove

- Facebook: www.facebook.com/pausefirstacademy

- Instagram: www.instagram.com/kimcolegrove_author/?hl=en

# Crisis Resources

**(If you or someone you know is in immediate danger, call 911 now)**

## FOR ALL FIRST RESPONDERS

### 988 Suicide and Crisis Hotline

- Nationwide, free, confidential support for people in distress.
- Dial 988

### Suicide.org

- Suicide prevention, awareness, and support.
- www.suicide.org
- 1-800-SUICIDE (1-800-784-2433)

### Crisis Text Line

- Connect with a volunteer crisis counselor by text, talk, or WhatsApp.
- Text HOME to 741741
- www.crisistextline.org

### Safe Call Now

- 24-hour confidential crisis referral service staffed by first responders.

- For public safety professionals, emergency services personnel, and family members.

- Assistance with treatment options for mental health, substance abuse and other personal issues.

- www.safecallnowusa.org

- 1-206-459-3020

# FOR LAW ENFORCEMENT

### Copline

- Law Enforcement Officer hotline for officers and their family members.

- Guarantees confidentiality and anonymity.

- Lines answered by trained, competent, retired officers.

- www.copline.org

- 1-800-267-5463

# FOR FIRE/EMS

### Fire/EMS Helpline

- Free, confidential.
- www.nvfc.org/helpline
- 1-888-731-3473

### Share the Load Program

- A behavioral health directory of resources.
- www.nvfc.org/help

# FOR VETERANS

### Veterans Crisis Line

- A 24/7 Confidential Crisis Line
- Call, text, or chat online
- Dial 988, then press 1
- Text 83825
- www.veteranscrisisline.net

# Resources

**Books, articles, podcasts, apps, and more
to help you begin your journey to well-being**

Welcome to the resource guide for *The Mindfulness for Warriors Handbook*, a comprehensive companion designed to support first responders' mental health and well-being. This guide provides a broad array of resources tailored to enhance your understanding of the book's themes, reinforce mindfulness practice, and offer further stress management and self-care tools.

First responders are known for their courage and dedication, often stepping into scenarios many of us can't imagine. However, this bravery doesn't make them immune to the mental and emotional toll their work can take. This resource guide is created with the understanding of the unique challenges faced by first responders. It offers a range of tools designed to provide support, foster resilience, and promote wellness, created by the Mango Publishing team with Kim's oversight and experience as a guide.

Here, you'll find:

- **Books:** An essential reading list to deepen your knowledge of stress management, mindfulness, and the unique experiences of first responders.

- **Articles:** Selected writings offering additional insights and up-to-date research relevant to first responders and their wellness journey.

- **Podcasts:** Thought-provoking and informative podcasts focused on first responder wellness, offering an opportunity to learn from experts and peers in your field.

- **Apps:** Hand-picked applications that are designed to support mental health, facilitate mindfulness, and relieve stress.

- **Websites/Blogs:** A collection of useful websites and blogs offering resources, personal experiences, advice, and the latest information on wellness and mindfulness.

- **Inspiring Talks:** Quick boosts of understanding and knowledge from scientists and fellow first responders.

- **Programs, Courses, and Workshops:** Options for in-person or virtual classes or programs for first responders seeking support.

- **Support Networks:** An array of support groups, community organizations, and online communities where first responders can connect, discuss, and provide mutual support.

- **Equipment/Tools:** Recommendations for equipment and tools that aid in practicing mindfulness, managing stress, and enhancing overall wellness.

The path of a first responder is undeniably challenging, but you're not alone on this journey. This guide is designed to be a beacon, lighting the way toward improved mental health, enhanced resilience, and a deeper understanding of the power of mindfulness. We invite you to explore these resources and integrate them into your journey toward wellness.

# BOOKS

Literature can be a profound source of inspiration, information, and guidance, especially in mental health, stress management, and resilience. This section introduces a selection of carefully curated readings that are especially pertinent to first responders. These works touch upon various themes, such as the impact of trauma on the mind and body, the art of cultivating resilience, and the importance of emotional intelligence. Whether you're interested in personal narratives, scientific research, or practical self-help guides, this list offers diverse insights that can enhance your well-being and professional practice.

- *10% Happier*—**Dan Harris**: A true story of a news anchor who found meditation after having a panic attack on live TV. He shares his journey and how meditation helped him reduce stress and improve his life.

- *The Body Keeps the Score*—**Bessel van der Kolk**: A book about how trauma affects the body and mind. It explains how trauma can cause physical and emotional problems and provides healing methods.

- *Bulletproof Spirit*—**Captain Dan Willis**: A book about developing resilience in adversity. It provides practical tips on how to overcome challenges and become more resilient.

- *Emotional Intelligence*—**Daniel Goleman**: A book about how emotional intelligence can help you succeed. It explains what emotional intelligence is, why it's essential, and how to develop it.

- *Emotional Survival for Law Enforcement*—**Kevin Gilmartin, PhD**: A book about how law enforcement officers can cope with the stress of their job. It provides practical tips on how to manage stress and maintain mental health.

- *First Responder Resilience*—**Tania Glenn**: A book about how first responders can develop resilience in adversity. It provides practical tips on how to overcome challenges and become more resilient.

- *I Love a Firefighter*—**Ellen Kirschman**: A book about how to cope with the unique challenges of being in a relationship with a firefighter. It provides practical tips on how to maintain a healthy relationship.

- *Increasing Resilience in Police and Emergency Personnel*—**Stephanie M. Conn**: A book about how police officers and emergency personnel can develop resilience in the face of adversity. It provides practical tips on how to overcome challenges and become more resilient.

- *Man's Search for Meaning*—**Viktor E. Frankl**: Although not specifically targeted at first responders, Frankl's classic work can provide profound insights on resilience and finding purpose in the midst of suffering, themes that may resonate with those in high-stress, trauma-exposed professions.

- *Mindsight*—**Dr. Daniel Siegel**: A book about how the mind works and how we can change it. It explains what mindsight is, why it's essential, and how to develop it.

- *The Power of Vulnerability*—**Brené Brown**: A book about how vulnerability can help us connect with others and live more fulfilling lives. It explains vulnerability, its importance, and how to embrace it.

- *Relentless Courage*—**Michael Sugrue & Shauna Springer, PhD**: A book about how veterans can overcome PTSD and other mental health issues. It provides practical tips on how to manage symptoms and improve mental health.

- *Resilient*—**Dr. Rick Hanson**: A book about how to develop resilience in the face of adversity. It provides practical tips on how to overcome challenges and become more resilient.

- *Trauma Stewardship*—**by Laura van Dernoot Lipsky**: This book offers practical tools for those who work to alleviate the suffering of others and could be very applicable for first responders.

- *The Upside of Stress*—**Kelly McGonigal**: A book about how stress can benefit us. It explains what stress is, why it's essential, and how we can use it to our advantage.

# ARTICLES

The following curated list of articles can significantly contribute to your knowledge about essential topics like mindfulness, stress management, the benefits of yoga and meditation, overcoming mental health stigmas, and trauma-informed leadership. Each article provides a unique perspective on the challenges first responders face, their mental health needs, and the practices they can adopt to lead healthier lives. This diverse collection aims to provide you with a comprehensive understanding of the subject, incorporating viewpoints from different authors, domains, and experiences.

Goerling, Richard. "The Case for Mindfulness in Policing." Calebrepress.com. May 23, 2018. www.calibrepress. com/2018/05/the-case-for-mindfulness-in-policing

Baum, Naomi L. "Demystifying Mindfulness." *Fire Rescue Magazine*. June 26, 2017. firerescuemagazine.firefighternation. com/2017/06/26/demystifying-mindfulness

McGreevey, Sue. "Eight Weeks to a Better Brain." *The Harvard Gazette*. January 21, 2011. news.harvard.edu/gazette/ story/2011/01/eight-weeks-to-a-better-brain

Luster, Rodney. "First Responders and Mental Health: When Heroes Need Rescuing." *Psychiatric Times*. September 9, 2022. www.psychiatrictimes.com/view/first-responders- and-mental-health-when-heroes-need-rescuing

Hummell, Wendy. "How yoga and meditation helped sharpen my aim." *Police1*. August 20, 2018. www.police1.com/police- training/articles/how-yoga-and-meditation-helped- sharpen-my-aim-U1igYyNBTQ1RSINh

Pittaro, Michael. "Mental Health Care for First Responders: Confronting the stigma and barriers to treatment." *Psychology Today*. July 3, 2019. www.psychologytoday.com/us/blog/ the-crime-and-justice-doctor/201907/mental-health-care- first-responders

Wolkin, Jennifer. "The Science of Trauma, Mindfulness, and PTSD." Mindful.org. June 15, 2016. www.mindful.org/the- science-of-trauma-mindfulness-ptsd

Bustos, Cathy. "Trauma-Informed Leadership." *Police Chief Magazine*. May 24, 2023. www.policechiefmagazine.org/ trauma-informed-leadership

# PODCASTS

Welcome to the podcast section of our resource guide. Podcasts are an excellent medium for learning, growth, and support, as they offer a unique blend of storytelling, expert insights, and actionable advice.

Our list encompasses podcasts that offer a broad perspective on the life and experiences of first responders. They delve into various topics, including mental health, physical fitness, resilience, leadership, stress management, and career development. Although not all these podcasts are tailored specifically for first responders, they present themes and discussions that can benefit their well-being and professional development.

- **The Guns and Yoga Podacast:** Host Wendy Hummell, a 25-year law enforcement professional and Yogi, examines all aspects of first responder wellness. Named a 2022 Top 12 podcast by PoliceOne.

- **The Squad Room:** This podcast is designed for law enforcement professionals. It explores mental health, physical fitness, leadership, and career development topics.

- **The Washdown Podcast:** Firefighters and other first responders discuss mental health, wellness and other topics of interest.

- **Alpha Human Podcast:** While not explicitly focused on first responders, this podcast shares stories of resilience, strength, and overcoming adversity—themes that can resonate with and inspire first responders.

- **Behind the Shield:** This podcast is designed for firefighters. It explores mental health, physical fitness, leadership, and career development topics.

- **Crisis Intervention Team Inc. Podcast:** Focused on reducing the stigma around mental health discussions, this podcast addresses specific issues first responders face, like PTSD, and presents various ways to manage these challenges.

- **Dear Chiefs Podcast:** This podcast is designed for fire service leaders. It offers insights into leadership, management, and organizational culture.

- **The First Responder Fitness Podcast:** A podcast dedicated to physical fitness and wellness strategies for first responders, offering ways to maintain optimal physical health while handling the high-stress environment of first responder work.

- **First Responder Trauma Counselors' Podcast:** This podcast explores mental health topics and trauma, especially those experienced by first responders, offering advice from professionals and sharing stories from other first responders.

- **Health, Nutrition, and Functional Medicine Podcast:** This podcast is designed to help first responders improve their health through nutrition and functional medicine. It offers insights into how nutrition can help manage stress and improve well-being.

- **Inside EMS Podcast:** A podcast for and about EMS professionals, discussing issues like mental health, job-related stress, and methods to cope with them. It also offers insights into the latest EMS news and trends.

- **Meditative Story**: Although not specifically for first responders, this podcast combines inspirational stories narrators tell with meditative music to induce a mindful state, potentially useful for relaxation and stress reduction.

- **The Mindful Badge Podcast**: This show focuses on the mental well-being of first responders, discussing various mindfulness and meditation techniques that can be incorporated into their daily routines to reduce stress and promote mental resilience.

- **No One Fights Alone:** This podcast is designed for first responders. It explores mental health, physical fitness, leadership, and career development topics.

- **Behind the Shield:** A mental health and support resource for emergency service professionals and their families from James Geering.

- **The Warrior Wellness Podcast:** This podcast is for military members, veterans, and first responders, focusing on fitness, health, nutrition, and biohacking. Its mission is to introduce America's heroes to lifestyle habits and hacks to help them live healthier, happier lives.

## APPS

As the world increasingly goes digital, our mental health support and resources have followed suit. Mobile applications have made wellness resources incredibly accessible, allowing us to engage in health-promoting activities like meditation, sleep management, stress reduction, and much more, right at our fingertips.

The apps listed below cater to various aspects of first responders' mental health and overall well-being. Some of these are designed explicitly with first responders in mind, while others address the broader themes of mental health, stress management, and mindfulness. Regardless of their specific focus, each of these apps offers valuable tools and strategies that can help first responders navigate their unique challenges. However, these apps are not a substitute for professional help when it is needed. They are part of a broader wellness strategy that includes professional mental health support, social connection, physical activity, and adequate rest.

- **10% Happier**: Based on the bestselling book by Dan Harris, this app offers a wide range of guided meditations, including courses specifically designed for coping with stress and anxiety.

- **Aura**: Provides mindfulness meditations, life coaching, stories, and music, all personalized based on the mood you select when you open the app.

- **Breathe2Relax**: This app provides detailed information on the effects of stress on the body and instructions on stress management exercises, such as diaphragmatic breathing.

- **Calm**: Calm is a leading app for meditation and sleep, offering guided meditations, Sleep Stories, breathing programs, stretching exercises, and relaxing music. The app is designed to help users reduce stress and anxiety, improve focus, and get better sleep.

- **Headspace**: Headspace offers guided meditations, animations, articles, and videos, all in the distinct Headspace style. The app covers topics like stress, sleep, focus, and anxiety, offering courses on mindful living and even workout routines.

- **Insight Timer**: This app features over 80,000 free guided meditations, music tracks, and talks from mindfulness experts. You can choose sessions according to your available time, varying from one minute to several hours. It also offers an advanced timer for silent meditations and bedtime stories to help you sleep.

- **Meditopia**: Meditopia is a meditation app that helps users reduce stress, sleep well, build mental resilience, and experience long-term relaxation. The app offers over a thousand guided meditations on stress, anxiety, happiness, self-love, focus, calm, and personal growth.

- **MyLife Meditation (formerly Stop, Breathe & Think)**: A meditation app that allows you to check in with your emotions and then recommends short, guided meditations, yoga, and acupressure videos, tuned to how you feel.

- **PTSD Coach**: Created by the Veterans Administration, PTSD Coach offers self-help strategies and resources to manage trauma-related symptoms.

- **Sanvello**: An app designed to help manage stress, anxiety, and depression through cognitive-behavioral therapy, mindfulness meditation, and other mental health practices.

- **Sleep Cycle**: Focused on improving sleep quality, the app analyzes sleep patterns and wakes users during their lightest sleep phase to ensure they wake feeling rested.

- **Smiling Mind**: A mindfulness app developed by psychologists and educators that offers a range of programs for all ages, including programs to assist with sleep, relationships, and performance.

- **Streaks**: Streaks is a to-do list that helps you form good habits. You can customize the app to help you maintain a streak in any activity, such as meditation, exercise, or reading. It's an excellent tool for motivating consistent behaviors that contribute to wellness.

- **The Resilience Project**: This app provides practical, evidence-based mental health strategies to build resilience and happiness. It offers activities to help you remain calm and mindful, develop gratitude and empathy, and increase emotional literacy.

- **Tide—Sleep & Meditation**: This app combines natural sounds with mindfulness practices to improve sleep, focus, relaxation, and meditation. It offers features like a focus timer, breathing guide, and meditation sessions.

## WEBSITES/BLOGS

In today's digital age, a wealth of knowledge and support is just a click away. Numerous websites and blogs provide valuable information, support, and resources for first responders and their families dealing with stress, trauma, and the unique challenges they face in their roles. These online platforms offer a range of insights—from expert advice and evidence-based strategies to personal stories of overcoming adversity.

Whether you are a first responder seeking coping strategies or a family member looking for understanding, these websites offer various perspectives and resources. We encourage you to explore these online spaces to deepen your understanding, find community, and discover helpful tools and techniques.

Please note that while we have taken care to include trusted and reliable sources, the content and views expressed on these websites are their own. Always consult with a healthcare professional for personal medical advice.

- **Pause First Academy** (www.pausefirst.com): This organization is owned and operated by Kim Colegrove. Visit the website to learn more about their in-person and online training. Visit the online academy to view on-demand courses and content created specifically for first responders. (Options available for individuals and organizations) (www.academy.pausefirst.com)

- **Firefighter Behavioral Health Alliance (FBHA)** (www. ffbha.org): This organization is dedicated to providing behavioral health workshops to fire departments and EMS organizations across the globe.

- **First Responder Wellness** (www.firstresponder-wellness. com/blog): This blog provides wellness resources specifically tailored to first responders, including mental health support and advice.

- **Headspace Blog** (www.headspace.com/blog): The blog of the popular meditation app focusing on mindfulness, meditation, and related topics.

- **Mindful** (www.mindful.org): This website is an excellent resource on mindfulness practices, research, and advice.

- **The Mindful Badge Initiative** (www.mindfulbadge. com): This organization provides mindfulness training specifically for law enforcement and first responders.

- **National Alliance on Mental Illness (NAMI) Blog** (www. nami.org/Blogs): The blog of NAMI provides a range of mental health resources, including posts focused on first responders.

- **PoliceOne** (www.policeone.com/health-fitness): This website is a comprehensive resource for law enforcement professionals, whose health and fitness section covers physical and mental well-being.

- **Psychology Today** (www.psychologytoday.com): Contains a vast range of articles from professionals about mental health, self-improvement, and behavioral science, including trauma and stress management.

- **The Resilience Project** (www.resilienceproject.com.au): A resource providing practical, evidence-based mental health strategies to build resilience.

- **Tema Conter Memorial Trust** (www.tema.ca): This Canadian organization provides resources for first responders dealing with mental stress and trauma.

# INSPIRATIONAL TALKS
# & MINDFUL DISCUSSIONS

- **"All It Takes Is 10 Mindful Minutes"** by Andy Puddicombe on TEDTalks: A brief, engaging talk about the value of taking a few minutes daily for mindful meditation.

- **"Building Resilience"** by Lucy Hone on TEDxChristchurch: This presentation discusses the strategies for building resilience in the face of adversity.

- **"Depression, the Secret We Share"** by Andrew Solomon on TEDTalks: A profound talk on understanding and coping with depression.

- **"Grit: The Power of Passion and Perseverance"** by Angela Lee Duckworth on TEDTalks: An insightful talk about the power of resilience and perseverance.

- **"How Mindfulness Changes the Emotional Life of Our Brains"** by Richard J. Davidson, on TEDxSanFrancisco: Renowned neuroscientist Richard J. Davidson discusses the impact of mindfulness on the brain's emotional response.

- **"Mindfulness and Neural Integration"** by Daniel Siegel, MD at TEDxStudioCityED: A discussion on how mindfulness impacts the brain and can lead to neural integration, improving mental health and well-being.

- **"The Power of Vulnerability"** by Brené Brown on TEDTalks: While not specific to first responders, this talk on vulnerability can benefit those dealing with emotional stress and trauma.

- **"Why We All Need to Practice Emotional First Aid"** by Guy Winch on TEDTalks: A TED talk focusing on the importance of taking care of our emotional health as we do our physical health.

- **"Yoga for First Responders"** by Olivia Kvitne Mead, YouTube: This is a quick introduction to the benefits of Yoga for First Responders by the program's founder.

# PROGRAMS, COURSES AND WORKSHOPS

- **The Battle Within** (thebattlewithin.org)—The program offers a five-day group therapy program created by fellow warriors to help others suffering from PTSD understand the traumas they have endured in service to others, provide an introduction to integrative tools that set the stage for healing, and develop a community of support. It also offers ninety-day classes built to fit into warriors' busy lives and provided by partner organizations that develop into habits the tools introduced during the Revenant Journey, such as fitness, equine, meditation, spiritual, nutrition, and arts programs.

- **West Coast Post-Trauma Retreat** (www.frsn.org/west-coast-post-trauma-retreat.html)— A residential program designed to help current and retired first responders regain control over their lives.

- **Firefighter Behavioral Health Alliance Workshops**— These workshops provide behavioral health workshops to firefighters, their families, and departments.

- **First Responders First** (firstrespondersfirst.com)— Veterans and first responders have designed the program for veterans and first responders struggling with primary mental health, trauma, PTSD, addiction, depression, and co-occurring disorders.

- **Help for Our Heroes** (helpforourheroes.com)—The program is designed to help veterans and first responders struggling with primary mental health, trauma, PTSD, addiction, depression, and co-occurring disorders.

- **Mental Health First Aid for Fire and EMS by The National Council for Behavioral Health**—This course helps fire and EMS personnel understand mental health and offers strategies to help those experiencing a mental health crisis.

- **Mindful Badge Initiative**—Offers mindfulness training for law enforcement and first responders.

- **Mindfulness-Based Stress Reduction (MBSR) Online Course by Palouse Mindfulness**—A free, internationally recognized program designed to assist people in dealing with physical and emotional stress.

- **The Resilient First Responder by Dr. Stephanie Conn**—Provides first responders with the knowledge, techniques, and skills to build resilience and prevent trauma.

- **Responder Resilience Training by Acadia Healthcare**—These are comprehensive programs designed to promote resiliency among first responders and healthcare professionals.

- **Save A Warrior** (saveawarrior.org)—The program offers a holistic approach to healing combat veterans and first responders who have PTSD. It includes peer-to-peer support groups, outdoor activities such as hiking and camping trips, and mindfulness meditation.

- **Stress Management and Resiliency Training (SMART) for First Responders**—This is a course offered by the Benson-Henry Institute for Mind Body Medicine that provides evidence-based strategies for stress management.

- **Veteran's PATH** (veteranspath.org)—The program offers mindfulness-based retreats for veterans and their families. It also offers online courses on mindfulness meditation and other topics related to mental health.

- **"Demystifying Meditation and Mindfulness for Criminal Justice Professionals"** with instructor Kim Colegrove— Available on the Justice Clearinghouse website: www. justiceclearinghouse.com/resource/demystifying-meditation-and-mindfulness-for-criminal-justice-professionals/

- **"Tools to Manage the Stress Response"** with instructor Wendy Hummell—On the Justice Clearinghouse website: www.justiceclearinghouse.com/resource/tools-to-manage-the-stress-response/

- **Yoga for First Responders (YFFR)**—YFFR offers yoga and mindfulness training designed to help first responders process stress, build resilience, and enhance job performance.

## CONFERENCES/EVENTS

- **First Responder Mental Health and Wellness Conference:** Hosted by the American Institute for First Responders, this conference focuses on the challenges first responders face, discussing the importance of mental health and well-being in these high-stress professions.

- **Global Resilience Summit:** This summit focuses on building resilience, a crucial trait for first responders. It often includes talks on mindfulness as a tool for resilience.

- **Heroes Health Symposium:** An event focused on health and wellness strategies for first responders and military personnel, often featuring discussions on mindfulness techniques.

- **1st Responder Conferences (www.1strc.org):** Nationwide conferences for first responders focused on the emotional, physical, and spiritual well-being of the public safety workforce.

- **International Conference on Mindfulness (ICM):** This annual event offers a platform for exchanging knowledge related to mindfulness techniques, practice, and research, often attracting professionals, educators, and practitioners from across the globe.

- **International Symposium for Contemplative Research (ISCR):** An interdisciplinary conference that brings together academics, educators, and practitioners to discuss the latest research in mindfulness and meditation.

- **Meditative Mindfulness Congress:** An international event focusing on meditation practices and their implementation in various fields, including high-stress professions.

- **Mindful Leadership Summit:** An event focusing on integrating mindfulness into leadership, beneficial for leaders in first responder organizations.

- **Mindful Society Conference:** This event explores the application of mindfulness in a wide range of societal sectors, including healthcare, education, and public safety.

- **Mindfulness Expo:** A significant event hosting various workshops, speakers, and vendors centered around mindfulness practices.

- **National Alliance on Mental Illness (NAMI) Conferences:** While these events cover a broad range of mental health topics, there are often sessions dedicated to the mental health and wellness of first responders, including mindfulness strategies.

- **Wisdom 2.0 Conference:** This conference brings together people from various disciplines to explore how we can live with mindfulness, wisdom, and compassion in the digital age.

# SUPPORT NETWORKS

A support network can serve as a lifeline for first responders, offering them a safe space to share their experiences, seek advice, and find comfort in knowing they are not alone. These platforms can be particularly beneficial for those dealing with stress, trauma, and other mental health issues common in high-pressure professions. Whether you're looking for an online forum, a face-to-face support group, or a community organization, you will find a resource here that can provide the support you need.

## Support Groups and Forums

- **First H.E.L.P.** (www.1sthelp.org): This organization is working to reduce mental health stigma for first responders through education and awareness.

- **American Foundation for Suicide Prevention (AFSP) Peer Support:** Connects individuals who have experienced a suicide loss.

- **EMDR International Association—Trauma Recovery Networks:** While not a traditional support group, these networks offer resources and connections for individuals interested in EMDR therapy, a treatment often used for PTSD.

- **Mindful Badge Initiative:** Offers mindfulness training and resources for law enforcement, including online support groups and sessions.

- **NAMI's Homefront:** An online and in-person educational program for families, caregivers, and friends of military service members and veterans dealing with mental health conditions.

- **National Police Suicide Foundation Support Groups:** This foundation offers various resources for police officers and their families, including support groups.

- **Online Grief Support Forums:** Online communities where people dealing with grief can share their experiences and support each other.

- **Survivors of Suicide Loss Support Groups:** These groups provide a comforting environment for individuals who have lost a loved one to suicide.

## Community Organizations

- **The Code Green Campaign:** A first responder-oriented mental health advocacy and education organization.

- **EMDR International Association (EMDRIA):** Promotes health and growth for individuals who have experienced trauma, including first responders, through Eye Movement Desensitization and Reprocessing (EMDR) therapy.

- **Firefighter Behavioral Health Alliance (FBHA):** Dedicated to educating emergency services personnel and their families about behavioral health issues including, but not limited to, depression, PTSD, and suicide ideation.

- **First Responder Support Network (FRSN):** Offers educational treatment programs for first responders and their families.

- **National Alliance on Mental Illness (NAMI):** Provides resources and support for those struggling with mental health issues, including a particular focus on first responders.

- **National Emergency Services Wellness Institute (NESWI):** Aims to improve the mental, physical, and spiritual well-being of emergency service professionals.

- **Tema Conter Memorial Trust:** Provides training and resources for public safety and military personnel dealing with occupational stress and PTSD.

## EQUIPMENT/TOOLS

As we delve into mindfulness and stress management, we must remember that some practical tools and resources can enhance our journey. Below, we've compiled a list of equipment and tools that could be instrumental in furthering your mindfulness practice.

- **Anti-Stress Comfort Wrap:** Heat this wrap in the microwave and then wrap it around your neck and shoulders for deep tissue relaxation.

- **Essential Oils/Diffuser:** Essential oils like lavender and chamomile can be calming and used with meditation and relaxation practices.

The Mindfulness for Warriors Handbook

- **Journal**: A mindfulness journal can help track progress and experiences during meditation and mindfulness exercises.

- **Meditation Cushion or Bench**: To ensure comfortable sitting during meditation practices.

- **Mindfulness Cards**: These cards provide prompts and exercises to help incorporate mindfulness into the daily routine.

- **Muse Headband**: A tool used for biofeedback during meditation. The headband gives real-time feedback on brain activity, heart rate, breathing, and body movements to assist in developing a consistent and effective meditation practice.

- **Noise-Canceling Headphones**: These can be useful for blocking out distractions during meditation or relaxation practices.

- **Weighted Blanket**: Some people find that using a weighted blanket can have a calming effect, reducing anxiety and promoting better sleep.

- **Yoga Mat**: Useful for practicing yoga and body scan meditation.

## FINAL THOUGHTS

Consider this guide not an end but a stepping stone in your wellness journey. We encourage you to delve into these resources, engage in the conversations they spark, and utilize the tools they provide. Your wellness is a continuous journey and each resource

# Acknowledgments

I would like to sincerely thank the ten people who contributed to this book by allowing me to interview them.

Justin, Brenda, Adam, Nate, Dawn, John, Wendy, Myrone, Angela, and Keith: your stories have touched lives and inspired others to seek healing. You will never know how many people you've helped or how many lives you've saved.

Thank you for being honest and vulnerable and for reaching back to help others.

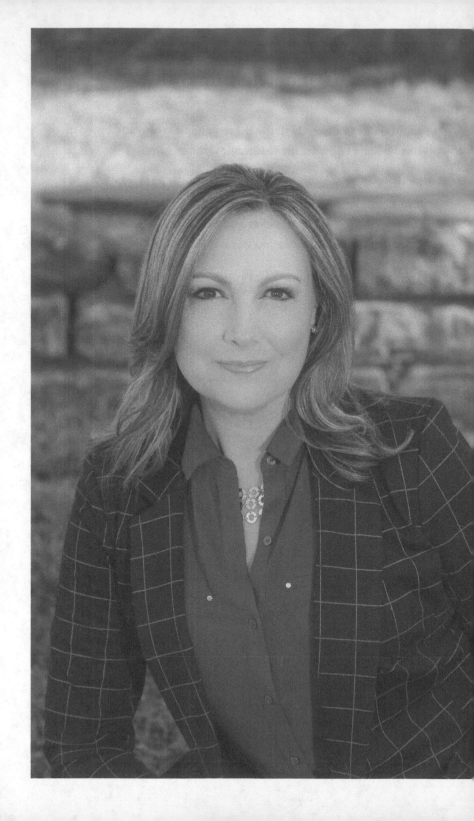

# About the Author

Kim Colegrove is a veteran meditator with over forty-five years of experience. She was originally trained in Transcendental Meditation at age ten. Although she no longer practices TM, she says it provided the foundation that helped her create the methodologies she uses to teach others about meditation.

In 2011, Kim left her corporate job to teach meditation and mindfulness full time. Initially, she taught small classes and worked with private clients, then transitioned to corporate settings. Her corporate clients include Garmin International, United Way, Department of Veterans Affairs, The National Court Reporters Association, and many others.

After losing her husband, former police officer and federal agent David Colegrove, to suicide, Kim turned her attention to first responders. She learned how prevalent chronic stress, anxiety, depression, silent suffering, and suicide are across first responder professions, and she wanted to do something to help.

She started writing on the topic of first responder mental and emotional health, developed curriculum for first responders, and created Pause First Academy—an organization that provides in-person and online wellness and resilience training for society's warriors, protectors, guardians, and healers.

Kim is an experienced keynote speaker and instructor, and in 2022 she was awarded the Mid-America CIT (Critical Incident Team) Teacher of the Year award. She and her team of culturally competent instructors work with first responders nationwide, speaking at conferences, offering continuing education and providing in-service training.

Individuals and organizations across the country are benefitting from Pause First Academy's Premier Membership, an online subscription service that delivers on-demand courses and content focused on wellness, resilience, and work-life balance.

Kim Colegrove's mission is to help normalize mental health support and wellness education for first responders by delivering information, education, and training.

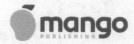

Mango Publishing, established in 2014, publishes an eclectic list of books by diverse authors—both new and established voices—on topics ranging from business, personal growth, women's empowerment, LGBTQ studies, health, and spirituality to history, popular culture, time management, decluttering, lifestyle, mental wellness, aging, and sustainable living. We were recently named 2019's #1 fastest growing independent publisher by *Publishers Weekly*. Our success is driven by our main goal, which is to publish high quality books that will entertain readers as well as make a positive difference in their lives.

Our readers are our most important resource; we value your input, suggestions, and ideas. We'd love to hear from you—after all, we are publishing books for you!

Please stay in touch with us and follow us at:

Facebook: Mango Publishing
Twitter: @MangoPublishing
Instagram: @MangoPublishing
LinkedIn: Mango Publishing
Pinterest: Mango Publishing

Sign up for our newsletter at www.mango.bz and receive a free book!

Join us on Mango's journey to reinvent publishing, one book at a time.

Printed in the USA
CPSIA information can be obtained
at www.ICGtesting.com
JSHW030301051023
R12986900002B/R129869PG49401JSX00001B/1